HEALING YOUR GRIEVING HEART WHEN SOMEONE YOU CARE ABOUT HAS ALZHEIMER'S

D1316901

12 -11

Also by Alan Wolfelt and Kirby Duvall:

Healing Your Grieving Body:
100 Physical Practices for Mourners

Healing After Job Loss:
100 Practical Ideas

Also by Alan Wolfelt:

Creating Meaningful Funeral Ceremonies:
A Guide for Families

Healing the Adult Child's Grieving Heart:
100 Practical Ideas After Your Parent Dies

Healing a Friend's Grieving Heart:
100 Practical Ideas for Helping Someone
You Love Through Loss

Healing Your Grieving Heart for Kids:
100 Practical Ideas

The Journey Through Grief:
Reflections on Healing

Understanding Your Grief:
Ten Essential Touchstones for Finding
Hope and Healing Your Heart

The Wilderness of Grief: Finding Your Way

Companion Press is dedicated to the education and support of both the bereaved and bereavement caregivers. We believe that those who companion the bereaved by walking with them as they journey in grief have a wondrous opportunity: to help others embrace and grow through grief—and to lead fuller, more deeply-lived lives themselves because of this important ministry.

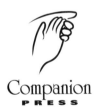

Companion
PRESS

For a complete catalog and ordering information, visit:

Companion Press
The Center for Loss and Life Transition
3735 Broken Bow Road
Fort Collins, CO 80526
(970) 226-6050
www.centerforloss.com

HEALING YOUR GRIEVING HEART WHEN SOMEONE YOU CARE ABOUT HAS ALZHEIMER'S

•

100 PRACTICAL IDEAS FOR FAMILIES, FRIENDS AND CAREGIVERS

•

ALAN D. WOLFELT, PH.D.
KIRBY J. DUVALL, M.D.

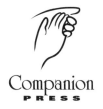

Companion
PRESS

Fort Collins, Colorado

An imprint of the Center for Loss and Life Transition

© 2011 by Alan D. Wolfelt, Ph.D. and Kirby J. Duvall, M.D.

All rights reserved. No part of this publication may be
reproduced, stored in a retrieval system, or transmitted
in any form or by any means, electronic, mechanical,
photocopying, recording or otherwise, without prior
permission of the publisher.

Companion Press is an imprint of the
Center for Loss and Life Transition,
3735 Broken Bow Road, Fort Collins, Colorado 80526
970-226-6050
www.centerforloss.com

Companion Press books may be purchased in bulk
for sales promotions, premiums or fundraisers. Please
contact the publisher at the above address for more
information.

Printed in the United States of America

16 15 14 13 12 11   5 4 3 2 1

ISBN: 978-1-617221-48-4

We dedicate this book in loving memory of our parents,
Donald and Virgene Wolfelt and Merle and Pauline Duvall,
whose love and support will always be with us.

INTRODUCTION

Someone you love has been diagnosed with Alzheimer's disease or dementia. You probably did not expect things to turn out this way. Emotionally, you may be finding it hard to accept the diagnosis even as you are caught up in planning for your loved one's present and future care. Of course, your own future is altered as well. All of this may seem overwhelming, but we have a hopeful message for you—a message that comes from our experiences working with Alzheimer's patients, families, and even our own parents:

You can and will survive this difficult time.

Our hope is that this book can be your companion as you navigate the sometimes treacherous and certainly emotion-packed journey of helping someone you love live with Alzheimer's. It is not an easy road. But loving someone with Alzheimer's does not necessarily mean that all is lost. By focusing on the abilities your loved one retains, you may still be able to have a meaningful relationship and share joy and love. And by fully mourning and making the most of your own days, despite the course of the disease, you will be living your life "on purpose," with meaning each and every day.

You are not alone

First of all, it's important to remember that you are not alone.

Today, about 5.3 million Americans are affected by Alzheimer's. The majority are 65 or older, but about five percent are diagnosed at younger ages. It is estimated that by the middle of the 21st century, three times this number of Americans will have Alzheimer's disease.

Who is caring for all these people? Currently, about 11 million U.S. family members and friends provide unpaid care for people with Alzheimer's disease. Their love, time, and attention help keep those affected by Alzheimer's safe and their lives meaningful. And even more families and friends are involved in helping to arrange this care, even though they may not be directly involved.

Whether you are a direct caregiver to someone with Alzheimer's or you are a family member or friend without daily caregiving responsibilities, this book is for you.

What is Alzheimer's?

Dementia is a nonspecific medical term for loss of mental functioning. The word literally comes from the Latin root meaning "without mind." It means loss or impairment of mental capabilities. It does not mean "crazy." It relates to a group of symptoms and is not the name of a disease that causes the symptoms.

There are several causes of dementia, including brain injury, stroke and other brain disease, but Alzheimer's disease is the most common type, accounting for somewhere around 60 to 80 percent of all cases of dementia. The remaining 20 to 40 percent are caused by diseases that rob the brain of oxygen, such as stroke, and other neurological disorders, such as Parkinson's disease. (Since Alzheimer's disease is the most common form of dementia, we primarily rely on that term throughout this book. However, if the person you love has a different or undifferentiated form of dementia, you will likely find that the content of this book is appropriate for you as well.)

Although we don't know exactly how Alzheimer's arises in the brain, we believe it involves the buildup of so-called plaques and tangles. Plaques are clumps of a protein called *beta-amyloid*, which starts to accumulate in the front of the brain and then gradually spreads to other parts. Tangles are twisted knots of another protein called *tau*, which arises from inside cells. Tangles start near the hippocampus, the brain's memory center, and then spread out from there.

A person's brain weighs only about three pounds, yet it is the most important part of the body. And when it is affected by Alzheimer's, the damage is progressive. Generally Alzheimer's is divided into an early-to-mild stage, a moderate stage, and a severe stage. The early-to-mild stage lasts around three to five years, during which time the brain damage is mainly in the memory areas. Because judgment, reasoning, and social skills are preserved, the person can develop compensatory coping strategies to deal with the memory problems. This disease's progression can last for up to 20 years, depending on the health and unique circumstances of the individual.

Memory loss in Alzheimer's disease

A slight forgetfulness is common as we age, but it usually does not interfere with our lives. However, severe memory loss is the hallmark of Alzheimer's disease.

The brain has multiple warehouses for storing memories. In early Alzheimer's the brain's temporary notepad, which retains information for a short time (like being able to remember directions to a gas station), still works, but there is trouble transferring this information to long-term storage due to brain damage at the hippocampus. Learning, math, drawing skills, and the person's sense of place, among other cognitive abilities, can also be affected.

Short-term memory soon becomes impaired by loss of episodic memory, which holds daily events. Both verbal memory—words you just heard—and visual memory—recognizing people and places—are lost. The person becomes more and more obviously confused.

Next affected is semantic memory, which is the memory of meanings and concepts as opposed to specific experiences. This information allows you to do your job and is dependent on your age and education. In Alzheimer's this type of memory falters only after episodic memory fails.

My Mother's Journey Through Dementia

In her younger days, Virgene Wolfelt was a very vital woman. She was a water-safety instructor trainer, a Cub Scout leader, and a mother of three busy children. You never had to guess about what was on her mind, because she would tell you—even if you didn't want to know it.

She was also a devoted wife to my father, who died four months after we celebrated their 50th wedding anniversary. For the next two years, Mom continued to function independently. She drove her car around town, bought her own groceries, and interacted with her many grandchildren. She lived at home by herself on five acres and was able to keep up with the demands of caring for herself and her home.

But then the changes started and never stopped. Poor judgment began to set in. She ordered a bicycle over the phone and crashed it the first time out. She began misplacing things and would become disoriented to time and place. She expressed a loss of initiative, often replying to our invitations, "I'll just stay home." She seemed to be aware that she was losing her mental capabilities, and she grew more quiet and withdrawn.

This is when I began to realize I would lose my mother twice—once to dementia and eventually to death.

I have to give Mom credit. While some people vigorously resist giving up their independence, Mom realized she could no longer live alone. She needed someone to help her remember to eat her meals and take her medications. I remember feeling so relieved that she was in a more structured environment and was safe and being cared for. I lived in Colorado, and she lived in Indiana. The distance never felt farther away.

As her dementia progressed, her personal care and grooming declined. She would often wear the same clothes each day and resisted changing into pajamas when it was time for bed. She didn't want to bathe or brush her teeth. Of course, she no longer had the capacity to manage her finances and make the simple decisions that before had come to her so easily.

At this point, Mom needed an even more structured care setting, so another move became necessary. And with that move came more changes, more losses, and more need for me to mourn the loss of my Mom as I once knew her. The smaller living space meant she had to give up more of her family's possessions, but she didn't seem to care. The photos, furniture, and other tangible symbols of my growing-up years were placed in storage.

As her dementia progressed, I watched Mom slip far away. She spent most of her time lying in bed. She needed constant care and had no desire to interact with the world around her. She lost track of who had visited her and when. One day after spending time with her, my brother called me and said that Mom wanted to know why it had been so long since I'd visited. Yet I had just been there, and my heart was broken to realize how far gone she was—from me and from all of us who loved her.

When she died on October 19, 2010, I was sad, but I was also relieved. She had lost her quality of life, and now I found peace in believing she had re-joined my father, the man she met on a school playground at the age of 14.

Yes, when someone we love has dementia, we grieve and we grieve and we grieve. We grieve the diagnosis, we grieve the many big and little losses along the way, and one day we grieve the death. I understand something of your journey, and I hope this book will be your companion as you learn to not only grieve but mourn. May you find joy and peace.

The next type of memory affected is procedural memory, which stores information below your awareness. It's the memory of how to do something almost automatically, such as play the piano. Early on, people with Alzheimer's may be able to make coffee in a coffee maker they've used for years but not be able to learn to use a new coffee maker. In later Alzheimer's even the old coffee pot may be confusing.

Long-term memory—things that happened at least two to five years ago—is somewhat resistant in Alzheimer's. People can often remember their first job, their mother's bedtime song, or something funny that happened in high school, yet they can't remember significant recent events, even major events like the death of a spouse. When this happens, you may find it very painful to have years or even decades of your shared history simply vanish.

But Alzheimer's is more than just memory loss. Your loved one has probably already shown some of the other early signs of the disease, including difficulty performing familiar tasks, language problems, disorientation to time and place, poor or worsening judgment, difficulties with abstract thinking, misplacing or losing things, changes in mood or behavior, personality changes, and even a loss of initiative.

As the disease progresses and more of the brain is affected, the person may begin to have problems getting dressed. He may become disoriented or lost in time. In the more severe stages, she may lose her ability to interact properly and may need nearly constant care. You may need help deciding when your loved one needs the around-the-clock care of an Alzheimer's unit or nursing home.

Caring for someone with Alzheimer's can be stressful. More than 40 percent of caregivers report a high or very high stress level. More than a third of caregivers report symptoms of depression. Relating to and caring for someone whose personality and moods are unpredictable can be overwhelming. And even if you do not have a direct caregiving role, you may still be overwhelmed by the stress of the changes.

Complicating the situation is the fact that families and friends often disagree about the best way to deal with the person with Alzheimer's. Some people will become only minimally involved yet want to make decisions, while others who are actually providing the care may feel overwhelmed by the work involved yet not able to have control of the situation. Longstanding family tensions can rise to the surface. Decisions about finances, the best course of treatment, the involvement of family, the use of respite care, and when and if to consider a nursing home or an Alzheimer's unit are all difficult questions to sort out.

You are experiencing loss, too

"My father started growing very quiet as Alzheimer's started claiming more of him. The early stages of Alzheimer's are the hardest because that person is aware that they're losing awareness. And I think that is why my father started growing more and more quiet."

- Patti Davis, daughter of Ronald Reagan

The progressive brain injury that occurs in Alzheimer's can slowly destroy function both physically and mentally. It is hard to watch as the losses accumulate and the person slowly loses awareness.

As the disease progresses, *you* also experience losses. Helping you acknowledge and mourn these losses is the subject of this book. You eventually lose the close personal relationship you had with the person you love. Your ability to do and enjoy the same things together is lost. Even the basis of the relationship may change. Role reversal is very common. Children of people with Alzheimer's have to act more like the parent. Most dramatically, your expected future has now been altered. You didn't plan for your life to turn out this way.

When we lose someone we care about and are attached to, we naturally grieve. As you experience the many losses that are part of loving someone with Alzheimer's, you too will grieve. But your grief may feel complicated. In some sense you need to mourn a person who is physically present but who is becoming more and more cognitively, emotionally, socially, and spiritually absent every day. Society, your friends, and even some of your family members may not understand this. This book will help you listen to your spirit and your own feelings and slow down to feel your inner pain. It will help you acknowledge and mourn what you have already lost and will be losing in the weeks and months to come. Finding ways to express what you feel on the inside is essential as you journey through the labyrinth that is Alzheimer's.

How this book is organized

To help enhance your understanding of your losses, we've divided this book into four sections:

- Acknowledge Your New Reality
- Allow Yourself to Mourn
- Join Your Loved One's New World
- Live with Meaning and Purpose

In the section entitled "Acknowledge Your New Reality," you'll find tips on how to come to terms with this difficult diagnosis and help yourself deal with the reality of your new situation. In the next section, "Allow Yourself to Mourn," you'll find suggestions on how to get in touch with the feelings you are having about the losses you are experiencing and encouragement to express them. Mourning is allowing the pain you are feeling inside to flow outward. In the section called "Join Your Loved One's New World" are ideas for focusing on the abilities that your loved one still has, despite the losses of Alzheimer's. The emphasis is on being aware of the presence of the person you love and joining him there whenever possible. In the last section, "Live with Meaning and Purpose," are ways for you to move forward with a sense of meaning and hope. Embracing what matters most to you and living your life as fully as possible will help you journey through grief and ultimately achieve not only reconciliation, but transformation.

As you move through the book, feel free to skip around, finding ideas that speak to you at this particular moment and ignoring those that don't. When you can, take advantage of the "Carpe Diems," which as fans of the movie *Dead Poets Society* will remember, means "seize the day." The Carpe Diem will help you achieve movement in your journey through grief right now, right this moment.

Our hope for you

We offer you this resource in an effort to help you with the natural challenges of loving someone who has Alzheimer's disease. In the months to come, you may experience what many people describe as "riding a roller-coaster of emotions." When faced with the ups and downs, you will be wise to remind yourself that despite the memory loss, lack of judgment, and personality changes exhibited by the person with dementia, he or she is still someone dear to you. You can continue to love your special person even as you begin to mourn the loss of him or her.

Yes, our hope is that this book can help you on this journey, but we realize it is no substitute for the help of so many others who are standing by to accompany you. The physicians, nurses, and other medical professionals who are trained to care for Alzheimer's patients will help. The social workers, therapists, and counselors who have experience working with families affected by Alzheimer's will help. Your family members, friends, and neighbors will help. Remember—*you need not walk this walk alone.* It is truly an honor for us to "companion" you at this difficult time of your life.

We hope to meet you one day.

Acknowledge your new reality

The first step on the road to healing your grief is to acknowledge your new reality. While at first feelings of shock, numbness, and denial are helpful—even necessary—in protecting you from the full force of your loss, you must slowly and in doses begin to accept both the diagnosis and your new reality. You must feel it to heal it.

1.

GENTLY EMBRACE THE REALITY THAT YOUR LOVED ONE HAS DEMENTIA OR ALZHEIMER'S

- For anyone experiencing the onset of dementia—the person affected as well as those who care about him—there is often an instinctual need to push away your new reality. You may be reluctant to consider Alzheimer's or even use the "A-word."

- Usually the onset of this disease is very subtle. Often only in retrospect do family members put the pieces together and recognize the disease's early symptoms.

- Your loved one may have experienced a string of tests trying to find something else that would account for her behavior changes. Since Alzheimer's disease is a clinical diagnosis with no one definitive test, it may have been difficult to reach this conclusion, with several doctors involved.

- You and your loved one may be understandably fearful to look into your shared future. You may not be able to accept this new reality all at once. But slowly, a little at a time, and as difficult as it is, you must mourn the loss of the future you expected and instead gently embrace your new reality. The first step in responding to this disease is acknowledging its day-to-day reality.

CARPE DIEM

Review the steps that have been taken to diagnose your loved one with Alzheimer's disease or dementia. Are you satisfied that this is the correct diagnosis? Reviewing the diagnosis one more time with the primary physician may help you begin to accept it. Getting another specialist's medical opinion may be needed for this acceptance to begin.

2.

RECOGNIZE THE
DIAGNOSIS AS A LOSS

- Someone you love has been diagnosed with dementia or Alzheimer's disease. This may feel overwhelming, both to you and to the person you love. You are both likely fearful of what the future holds.

- Your loved one has probably already had some memory problems, grown more easily confused, and even gotten lost in familiar places. You may have noticed personality changes, frustration in doing simple tasks, and obsessive worry or repetitive questions or actions.

- These losses are a result of a brain disease that first strikes the memory center then progresses to other parts of the brain, resulting in increasingly diminished cognitive ability.

- As the person you love experiences each new loss, you also have a corresponding loss. You lose a part of the person you loved and a part of the relationship you had. You may progressively lose your personal closeness, the understanding you had between you, and even the activities and human interactions you enjoyed together.

- Even though your loved one is still alive, you are already beginning to feel the loss.

CARPE DIEM

Make a list of the losses, big and small, that you have
already experienced since the person you love began to
be affected by dementia or Alzheimer's disease.

3.

UNDERSTAND GRIEF AS A PART OF LOSS

- Grief is a word we usually think of in association with the death of someone we love. But actually, grief follows every significant loss in our lives. The losses you are experiencing as a result of your loved one's illness certainly cause you to grieve, too.

- We grieve when we lose something we value, someone we care about. With grief comes a wide range of emotions. Shock, numbness, confusion, anxiety, guilt and regret are common. Anger, blame, resentment, sadness and sometimes relief are also often part of grief. These feelings may arise one at a time or, more typically, may blend together in a kind of ever-changing grief stew.

- In the days after your loved one's diagnosis of Alzheimer's, the pain you feel may be ever-present. It's OK to escape for a few hours each day and take a break from your feelings. You could seek refuge by going for a walk, reading a book, watching a movie, spending time with family, exercising, or having coffee with a supportive friend.

CARPE DIEM

Today, do something that brings you comfort. Maybe it's working in the garden, baking a pie, taking a long bath, or sitting by the fire. What comforts you? Indulge yourself with a comfort break today.

4.

KNOW THE COMMON
SYMPTOMS OF GRIEF

- Symptoms of grief can vary widely among those who love someone with Alzheimer's, but common ones include:
    - denial that the person you love is ill
    - periods of helplessness, despair, and depression
    - changes in appetite or sleeping patterns
    - feelings of anger or frustration toward the person with Alzheimer's
    - withdrawal from social activities, friends, family, and even the person with Alzheimer's
    - feelings of anxiety or confusion

- Especially if you are the primary caregiver, you may be too busy and feel too overwhelmed to recognize that you are grieving the slow loss of your loved one. You may just pass it off as just being down or stressed from the situation. Recognize that you are in grief and need to allow yourself to actively mourn.

- Allow yourself to feel and express the pain of your loss, in doses.

CARPE DIEM

Which grief symptoms have you experienced so far? Take time today to relieve these symptoms by doing something you enjoy.

5.

RECOGNIZE FEELINGS OF SHOCK, NUMBNESS, AND DISBELIEF

- You may find yourself not feeling much of anything. If so, you may be in shock. Feelings of shock, numbness, and disbelief are common, especially early after the diagnosis of Alzheimer's or dementia.

- These feelings are nature's way of protecting you from the full reality of your loss. Like anesthesia, they help you survive the pain of early grief. If this diagnosis shocked you to your core, it may be a blessing to feel numb.

- You may think, "I'll wake up and this will not have happened." Early grief is like a dream. Your emotions need time to catch up with what your mind has been told. Your body slows in response to this emotional shock, and you may not feel like doing anything.

- Feelings of passivity often go hand-in-hand with numbness. You may feel childlike or even neglect basic needs, like food, water, and sleep. Simple decisions may be hard when you are in shock. If your friends or family urge you to make decisions when you are experiencing shock, tell them you need time to absorb your new reality before you can think further ahead.

CARPE DIEM

If you are feeling numb, cancel any commitments that require concentration and decision-making. Let yourself regroup. Find a safe haven where you can retreat for a few days or for a few hours each day.

6.

BE IN TOUCH WITH YOUR BODY

- When we are grieving, we often feel bad physically. We may feel fatigue, headaches, stress, high blood pressure, and even body aches and pains. These symptoms are messages telling us that we need to slow down and turn inward to our grief.

- If you are in shock, your body will naturally slow down and your senses will be numbed. Your body is wise in this slowing. Well-intentioned people may divert you from honoring this slow-down. Society expects you to take just a day or two to regroup and then carry on dealing with the disease and your life. Ignore these expectations and go at your own pace.

- Stay in the present and focus on what you need to get through today rather than worrying about tomorrow. Just "being" may be all you are up to right now.

- Take care of your body. Say to yourself, "Right now I just need to breathe in and breathe out." Get plenty of rest, eat healthy foods, drink plenty of fluids, and walk or exercise if you are up to it. Make sure you are getting regular check-ups and medical care yourself.

- If you are the sole or main caregiver to someone who needs around-the-clock care or supervision, ask for occasional help. You cannot take care of your own health if you are constantly caring for someone else.

CARPE DIEM

Right now, sit in a comfortable position. Take ten deep, slow breaths—filling and emptying your lungs completely. When you finish, consider the essentials of what you need to do to get through this day. Just this day.

7.

BE GENTLE WITH YOURSELF AS YOU EXPERIENCE THE REPEATED LOSSES OF ALZHEIMER'S

"I'm in awe of people who deal with Alzheimer's, because they have to deal with death 10 times over, year after year."

– Maria Wallace

- Just as when you lose someone to death or divorce, you also feel loss when someone you love has Alzheimer's. But unlike a death, the advancing brain disease causes repeated and progressive losses.

- You lose the person you love a bit at a time. Like slowly removing a bandaid, it can seem more painful than one quick loss.

- With Alzheimer's, early losses often include the loss of the status quo of your relationship. There may be a painful redefinition of the relationships between parent and children, husband and wife. Have you already lost a sense of what is normal?

- As the disease progresses, caretaking becomes a full-time job, and if you are the primary caregiver, you may lose other parts of your life, including much of your free time and social life. The behavior changes of Alzheimer's may make caregiving difficult, and you may ultimately feel the loss of the close, loving relationship you once had.

CARPE DIEM

Be compassionate with yourself as you
struggle with a new aspect of loss.

8.

RECOGNIZE THE UNCERTAINTY IN YOUR LOSSES

"I often hear people say that the person suffering from Alzheimer's is not the person they knew. I wonder to myself, 'Who is he then?'"

– Bob DeMarco

• Everyone who loves someone with a debilitating and fatal disease experiences loss. We call the type of grief that comes with a terminal cancer diagnosis, for example, anticipatory grief, because it encompasses all the losses experienced on the journey as well as the anticipated death. When someone you love has dementia, you too experience a form of anticipatory grief, but yours may extend over a longer period of time (for some, as long as 20 years) and be socially unrecognized and surrounded by uncertainty.

• Psychologists call losses with some degree of uncertainty "ambiguous losses." As a caregiver, companion, or family member, you are faced with the loss of someone who is physically present but psychologically absent. What was once normal is now changed in your relationship.

• You may feel, "This is not my husband even though he looks like my husband" or, "My mother would never act like this." Even with the person present, your old relationship is engulfed in change. The grief you feel is naturally complicated by this ambiguity.

• To experience emotional and spiritual distress when confronted with the chronic illness of someone you love is very appropriate and understandable.

CARPE DIEM

Have you had any times of confusion or ambiguous feelings since your loved one was diagnosed with Alzheimer's? List them. Do you feel grief over these ambiguous and uncertain losses? Write your feelings down on paper.

9.

RESPOND TO FEELINGS
OF HELPLESSNESS

- It is not uncommon for family members to feel helpless, discouraged, or demoralized in the face of dementia. These feelings can be made worse if doctors or other professionals are not understanding and empathetic.

- But you have many resources within you. Although you cannot control or cure the disease, you can learn to shape your experience of it:

  - Take one day at a time.
  - Things seem worse when you focus on everything at once. Instead, focus on small things that you can change to improve life today.
  - Be informed about the disease. Read and learn from others about managing challenges.
  - Talk with families who face similar problems. Maybe join a support group.
  - Get involved in exchanging information, reaching out to others, or even supporting research.
  - Discuss your feelings with a doctor, social worker, psychologist, or clergyperson.
  - Maintain some personal hobbies and interests.
  - Eat healthy foods.
  - Get daily exercise, if only a 20-30-minute walk.

CARPE DIEM

Talk with someone close to you if you are feeling helpless.
Focus on a single, simple idea to make your life easier
or better. Having one success can lead to others.

10.

ASK FOR HELP

- When you experience a major loss, you need love and support from others. As you experience the cumulative losses that result from dementia or Alzheimer's disease, you especially need and deserve ongoing love and support. You may also need help just getting through each day if you are a caregiver.

- Don't feel ashamed of your heightened dependence on others right now. Don't expect yourself to do everything for your loved one or to handle your sense of grief and loss alone. You may need to talk this through with others. You may also need help with chores at home, medical appointments, or finances. Take comfort in the thought that others care about you and are available to help.

- Don't hesitate. Ask your friends and family for their support and patience. Those who love and care for you truly want to help. You just need to ask. Tell them specifically which tasks or chores they can do to help you right now. Also share with them how they can best help you process your emotions and acknowledge your loss.

- You can also phone the Alzheimer's Disease Education and Referral Center at no charge. The phone number is 1-800-438-4380. Or get help from them online at www.nia.nih.gov/Alzheimers.

CARPE DIEM

Call your closest friend right now and tell her you will need her help through the coming weeks and months. Ask her to be on call for you. You may need to meet weekly with her to laugh together or to have her listen to your frustrations.

11.

WATCH OUT FOR DEPRESSION

- Feeling down or blue is normal in dealing with significant problems like Alzheimer's. But if your depressed mood lasts longer than two or three weeks, or your feelings of anger, sadness, or hopelessness are getting worse, consider professional help.

- Ask yourself the following questions to determine if you could have depression:
    - Do I have little interest in things that are normally pleasurable?
    - Am I feeling down or depressed most of the time?
    - Am I having trouble falling or staying asleep?
    - Is my energy level low, leaving me feeling fatigued most of the time?
    - Has my appetite changed significantly?
    - Do I feel like a failure or guilty for no reason?
    - Am I having trouble concentrating and thinking clearly?
    - Am I moving more slowly or feeling more fidgety?
    - Am I feeling hopeless or even thinking about suicide?

- A "yes" answer to a few of these would be expected from the stress of dealing with Alzheimer's. But if you have positive answers to more than a few, it's time to seek help. Call a friend or meet with him to figure out a plan to deal with your depression. Or make an appointment with a primary care physician or counselor today.

CARPE DIEM

Consider how you feel right now. If are feeling depressed and have felt this way for some time, make a call for help. If you are temporarily feeling blue, do something positive to improve your mood.

12.

BE AWARE OF APATHY
AND NUMBNESS

- One of the most common traits of Alzheimer's is apathy, or loss of motivation, and this condition seems to have a biologic basis.

- Using brain scans, researchers report that changes in the brain's white matter in the frontal lobes are a common feature in apathetic Alzheimer's patients. Just over half of people with Alzheimer's are emotionally blunted and lack motivation and initiative.

- They may also withdraw from social contact as well as other activities. The symptoms resemble depression, but apathetic people have emotional indifference rather than the sadness, hopelessness, and guilt or shame of depression.

- When you are grieving, a similar symptom you may experience is numbness. It's common for people coping with the extended illness of someone they love to feel numb and emotionally flat at some point in their journey.

- It's important to rule out depression first, both for you and the person with Alzheimer's. True depression is associated with a chemical imbalance that can be treated.

- After depression has been ruled out or treated, combat apathy and numbness with activities that waken the senses. Go swimming. Build a snowman. Remain involved with others. Sample an ethnic cuisine you've never tried before.

CARPE DIEM

A life of apathy and numbness is a life without joy. When you're grieving, it's normal and natural to feel numb sometimes, but extended periods of numbness mean you probably need help. If this describes you, talk to your physician or try seeing a counselor for a few sessions.

13.

BE KIND TO YOURSELF

- You are going through a lot and you deserve kindness—from others but also from yourself.

- Maybe you have the urge to beat yourself up for what you have done, or failed to do, in dealing with your loved one's Alzheimer's. Let go of this self-doubt. You don't have to carry it with you. You are doing the best you can.

- Try being your own cheerleader. Get some sticky notes and write down a few phrases that have meaning for you, like "I am strong," "I can get through this," "I am doing the best I can," "While I'm not perfect, that is OK," "I cannot control some things," "What I'm experiencing would be difficult for anyone," then put them someplace where you will see them several times a day, like the bathroom mirror or the refrigerator.

- Celebrate even small successes. If you are the primary caregiver, say "Good job!" out loud to yourself when you are able to successfully get your loved one dressed with no emotional outbursts. If you are a friend or family member who does not have day-to-day caregiving responsibilities, pat yourself on the back whenever you reach out to offer your help and love.

CARPE DIEM

What are you beating yourself up about these days? Instead of being unkind to yourself, try this visualization. See yourself sitting on the bed, crying and feeling pain. Now see yourself sitting next to yourself and putting your arm around the other you's shoulder. Give her a hug. Rub her back as she cries. Sit together for a while.

14.

KEEP IT SIMPLE

• Your plate is likely very full in this trying time. If you are the primary caregiver to the person with Alzheimer's, you may feel emotionally, spiritually, and physically drained. If you are not the primary caregiver, you may have many other obligations and demands that are made more burdensome by your normal and natural grief.

• Keep your life simple right now. Do what you need to do to get through the day. Live moment-to-moment or hour-to-hour. Cancel unnecessary obligations; minimize nonessential chores and tasks.

• Spend any time you can with people you love doing things that give you pleasure. Eliminate or set limits on friends who drain you or make you feel worse.

• If you can, find a way to get out of the house. If you are feeling claustrophobic and stuck, get out and do something fun. If you are the primary caregiver, find someone who can take over your caregiving chores so you can have a break or maybe even a mini-vacation. Take a stroll in the woods, go for a walk with the dog, or peruse the shelves at a bookstore. It doesn't have to be a big event to help relieve your stress.

• Remember, it's OK to ask for help from family, friends, and others. You do not have to do everything yourself!

CARPE DIEM

Is there a commitment in your life that feels like a burden?
Maybe it is a monthly club meeting or a volunteer position.
Consider giving it up and de-stressing your schedule.

15.

UNDERSTAND THAT THE PERSON WITH DEMENTIA ISN'T "CRAZY"

- Through advances in science and brain imaging, we now understand that mental illness is the result of physical and chemical problems in the brain. Some of these differences we can see (for example, schizophrenics have larger brain ventricles than others); some we may not be able to (for example, the brain chemistry imbalances that create various psychiatric problems).

- So, dementia and Alzheimer's have a lot in common with mental illness. Both are diseases of the brain. You will probably notice that some of the typical behaviors associated with Alzheimer's—depression, irritability, aggression, paranoia—can also "look" and "sound" like mental illness.

- What we're hoping everyone keeps in mind is that, practically speaking, it doesn't matter whether or not Alzheimer's is a form of mental illness. When we use the term "crazy," we marginalize people with a very real physical problem. People who need our compassion and support. People who need our love and acceptance.

CARPE DIEM

The next time you catch yourself thinking that someone is "crazy," observe how the term makes you feel about the person. Try switching your perception from "crazy" to "disease" and notice if you feel differently.

16.

RECOGNIZE YOU'RE NOT CRAZY, EITHER

- When you love someone who has Alzheimer's, you might find your mind playing tricks on you.

- Both Alzheimer's disease and grief can feel like a trip into Alice's Wonderland, where nothing makes sense and reality seems distorted—sometimes mildly, sometimes beyond recognition.

- Did he really just say that? Did she actually just do that? The behaviors of a person affected by Alzheimer's can be so off-the-grid that you might find yourself questioning your own perceptions.

- Your natural grief and fatigue at this time will likely compound any feelings of confusion or disorientation you're experiencing as you watch the disease manifest.

- You're not crazy, either—you're mourning. Be gentle with yourself as well as with the person who has Alzheimer's.

CARPE DIEM

Talk to someone today about any feeling of disorientation or confusion you may be experiencing. A support group made up of others struggling with dementia in their family is a good place to voice these feelings. They will understand.

17.

HELP DISPEL OTHER MISCONCEPTIONS ABOUT ALZHEIMER'S

- Because of their close association with mental illness, dementia and Alzheimer's disease are surrounded by stigma and misconceptions.

- If you feel a sense of shame that someone you love has dementia, you have been affected by the stigma of Alzheimer's. Of course, the stigma implies that you or the person with the disease did something wrong, something that caused the problem or made it worse. Yet you are not to blame; nor is she.

- Educate yourself about the common myths by visiting the Alzheimer's Association website (alz.org). For example, you may have heard that drinking from aluminum cans and cooking in aluminum pots can lead to Alzheimer's disease, but studies have shown this isn't true.

- Talking with others who are knowledgeable about Alzheimer's and whose lives are also affected by it will help. Open communication is the antidote to harmful myths.

CARPE DIEM

Visit www.alz.org right now and do a search for the term "myths."
You'll find a list of common Alzheimer's misconceptions.

18.

TURN THE PAGE ON YOUR CALENDAR

- When someone loved is diagnosed with dementia or Alzheimer's, there is only Before and After. There is your life Before the diagnosis and now there is your life After. It's as if your internal calendar gets reset to mark the significance of the profound change.

- You may have experienced a similar phenomenon with other significant events in your life, such as getting married, having a child, or experiencing the death of someone you love. Each of these rites of passage marks a new season of your life. Your new season includes the presence-and-yet-absence of someone you love.

- If you are the primary caregiver, your life calendar may now involve challenging physical care as well as a host of other new tasks and limitations. Acknowledging your losses and seeing your current situation as a page in the calendar of your life may help you realize that this too shall pass.

CARPE DIEM

Write two columns on a piece of paper: Before and After.
In ten minutes, brainstorm as many adjectives or feelings
that you can think of that define each time period.

19.

EMBRACE YOUR UNIQUE STORY

- This book is intended to help support those grieving the progressive loss of someone they love to Alzheimer's disease or dementia. It addresses many of the common thoughts, feelings, and challenges you might experience.

- Yet grief is never one-size-fits-all. The losses you will confront as a result of this disease are uniquely yours, shaped by many influences. These include the relationship you have with the person who is ill, the circumstances you are both in, your personality, his personality, your history of loss, your culture and religious background, and many others.

- While you will likely find comfort and affirmation in sharing your story with others—especially people who have also loved and cared for someone with Alzheimer's, you will not always feel the same way they do. Unless you have lived their life and they have lived yours (which is, of course, not possible), you can never completely understand another's reality.

- You are unique. Your story of love and loss and grief and mourning is unique. Embrace this uniqueness and encourage others to embrace theirs.

CARPE DIEM

Right now, take a few minutes to make a list—in your
mind or on paper—of the ways in which your journey
through Alzheimer's grief is uniquely yours.

ALLOW YOURSELF TO MOURN

To mourn is to acknowledge what you feel on the inside and express it on the outside. Mourning can be difficult, especially if you're someone who has learned to "stuff" his or her feelings. Yet it is through mourning that grief is transformed into courage, hope, and love.

20.

GET YOUR GRIEF OUT

- Grief is the constellation of internal feelings and thoughts you experience with loss. Mourning, on the other hand, is external. It is the actions and words you use to express your grief. Mourning is grief gone public.

- You are grieving the slow, step-wise loss of your loved one from Alzheimer's. But to move through your loss, you must also mourn. If you grieve but don't mourn, you will likely get stuck in depression, anger, or fear. Besides depression, unexpressed grief can cause headaches, fatigue, stomachaches, and trouble sleeping.

- We all know that when we avoid our feelings, they usually come out in some unintended way. Stuffing our feelings can cause us to be impatient with those around us, irritated by even small inconveniences, or tearful for no apparent reason.

- Open yourself up and give yourself permission to mourn. Allow yourself to cry, talk, write, or even let out a scream when no one is around. Whatever it takes, do it. Get your grief out. When you do, you'll feel yourself begin to move through it and come back into your life again.

CARPE DIEM

Tell your story of Alzheimer's-related loss to someone today. Telling your story over and over again is like taking a shower every day. It washes away the grit and grime for a while. Eventually, the telling will get less and less painful and hold less emotional charge for you.

21.

RECOGNIZE THAT YOUR FEELINGS ARE IMPORTANT

- Our feelings are what make us human. We like to say that our feelings are the voice of our soul.

- Sometimes one feeling, like kindness, may surface. But at other times you may experience a rush of mixed feelings, especially in stressful situations. You might feel anxious, fearful, disrespected, and frustrated, all at the same time.

- As they grow up, some people are taught (usually subconsciously) to hide their feelings from others. Often they end up hiding them from themselves. This habit can make their emotional reactions a puzzle to themselves and others. If this sounds like you, you might have to make a conscious effort to recognize your own feelings. What is it you are feeling right now?

- Honor your feelings, even when they seem "negative." Remember that no feeling is right or wrong, it just is. Keep in mind that emotions need motion!

- Experiencing your authentic emotions allows them to flow through you in ways that create change and movement. Denying you are sad, for example, doesn't make it go away, but expressing it can help soften it.

CARPE DIEM

Right now, close your eyes and focus on breathing in and out to a count of 100. Then ask yourself: What am I feeling right now?

22.

NAME YOUR FEELINGS

- It's normal to be confused by multiple emotions during times of transition. Anger, worry, guilt, worthlessness, and despair may all be present. You may feel lost and alone. You may feel out of sync and separated from others. Or you may be overwhelmed by emotion and unsure of what you are feeling.

- Sometimes emotions come in waves, making them difficult to identify. Learning to name your emotions helps you tame them. As Shakespeare's Macbeth said, "Give sorrow words: the sorrow that does not speak whispers with o'er fraught heart, and bids it to break."

- Try a few ways to identify what it is you are feeling. Here are some examples:

  - Crank up the music, listen, and express yourself by yelling or singing along loudly. See what emotions arise.
  - Give yourself a voice. Try to evoke your feelings by saying, "I feel angry today because…." or "I could cry today about…"
  - Ask yourself what you are feeling while driving in the car, taking a shower, or right after you wake up. These are times when unfettered feelings may surface.

CARPE DIEM

Try writing a letter to your loved one expressing what you are feeling right now about her Alzheimer's. You don't have to send or show her the letter. Simply use it as a way to name your emotions.

23.

LEAN INTO YOUR GRIEF

- Stay in touch with your feelings by leaning into them when you can. Practically, this means when feelings come up, stop and feel them. Share them with a friend or write them down. Doing so can help release your grief.

- Generally we have been taught that emotional pain is to be avoided, not embraced. However, it is only in moving toward pain and grief that we can heal our wounds.

- Be wary if others are telling you how well you are doing with your "situation" or if you are not feeling much at all. Sometimes doing well means you are avoiding your pain, hiding your emotions, or experiencing some of the natural numbness that grief brings.

- Of course, it is important to pace yourself when you are allowing your grief and pain to surface. Sometimes you will need distractions from the pain, so you can set it aside for a bit and move through your day. This is called dosing yourself with your grief.

- As Helen Keller once said, "The only way to the other side of something is through it." Practice moving through your grief and pain rather than trying to go around it or ignore its presence.

CARPE DIEM

Today, find someone to talk with. Share your thoughts and emotions about the losses you have felt since the person you love began to be affected by Alzheimer's.

24.

BREAK DOWN ISOLATION

- Sometimes the primary caregiver to the person with Alzheimer's feels that he or she is facing this disease alone. If you are the husband or wife of someone with Alzheimer's, you may feel despair and loneliness because the one person with whom you could share your life is no longer able to be your close friend and confidant.

- Friends and family members who are not the primary caregiver to the person who has Alzheimer's may also feel isolated. You may feel that you are no longer a part of the person's life. If you don't personally know others whose lives are affected by Alzheimer's, you may also feel alone as you struggle to cope with your feelings of grief.

- Remaining involved with others—your family, friends, others who have family members with Alzheimer's—can help you feel less alone. Share your experiences with them, let them know how you feel. They may well have similar thoughts, feelings, and experiences.

- While you can never replace the relationship you had with the person affected by Alzheimer's, you will find that you do have friends and family who will offer you love and support if you only ask for it.

CARPE DIEM

Take a moment and find a quiet place to sit. Visualize your loved one standing beside you and hugging you for the care you show him. Visualize your friends behind you stepping up to hug and pull you closer. Recognize and process that your loved one both loves and appreciates you and that your friends will support you and pull you closer if you only reach out to them.

25.

ACKNOWLEDGE THAT MOURNING CAN BE COMPLICATED IN ALZHEIMER'S

- In tribal societies, and even in our own Western society of the past, loss and life transitions were marked by ritual and an outward display of emotions. Mourners used to dress in black, for example, as an outward sign of their loss.

- But with our fast-paced, highly technical, socially mobile, secularized and de-ritualized modern society, even the mourning of death seems at times to be slighted. Many people are choosing to have "celebrations" or "parties" instead of authentic funerals.

- But we, as humans, need to show outwardly how we feel in order to mourn our losses. Furthermore, mourning in Alzheimer's is not only complicated by the trends of modern society, it is further complicated by the fact the person is still alive. Others may not recognize your many losses along the way.

- If you are caring for a person with Alzheimer's, expect to have continued and ever-changing feelings of loss and grief as your life and the person you love are changed by the disease. These feelings are difficult, but they are normal. Everyone grieves differently and at his or her own pace. If your grief is so intense that your wellbeing is at risk, don't be afraid to ask for help from your doctor or a professional counselor.

CARPE DIEM

What complications do you see in trying to mourn your losses? Write them down. How can you get around these complications to show your painful feelings outwardly?

26.

FEEL YOUR PAIN, BUT IN DOSES

- Embracing painful emotions is not something that anyone wants to do. Why feel pain? It hurts, and it's hard to do! Avoiding, repressing, or pushing away your pain is easier to do than confronting and embracing it.

- Recognize that you must befriend your feelings, whatever they are, in small doses over time. Ask yourself how you feel about the losses from Alzheimer's and write down or share what comes up—then take a break. You can't take in the enormity of your losses all at once. It is healthy to seek distraction and take breaks for pleasure and comfort each day.

- Consider whether you are distracting yourself from your true feelings too much, however. Are you too busy with caregiving to feel anything? Do you avoid your feelings even when you have time? Make a conscious effort to make time to allow your deepest emotions to surface, a little at a time. They will probably keep trying to get your attention until you them the attention they demand and deserve.

CARPE DIEM

Take a walk, ride a bike, or go to the gym. Doing something physical can help you release your emotions. Or do the opposite and sit in silence. Listen to the birds, watch the trees sway in the wind. When feelings come up, feel them. Don't push them away or use reason to avoid them. Take a little time each day to feel your feelings.

27.

GET ENOUGH SLEEP

- You simply can't be healthy—physically, emotionally, or spiritually—if you're not getting enough sleep. Remember—when you are unable to get enough sleep, your fatigue will make any feelings of helplessness and discouragement you may have even worse.

- If you're struggling with losing someone you love to Alzheimer's, your grief is exhausting enough. It's like a demanding toddler who needs your attention. And as those of us who are parents know, it's really hard to take care of a toddler if you're sleep-deprived.

- If you're the primary caregiver to the person with Alzheimer's, not getting enough sleep is doubly problematic because the person may need as much care as a child, which is incredibly fatiguing, AND your grief also needs you.

- Then there's the fact that people with Alzheimer's often have disrupted sleep patterns that cause them to wake up and wander at night.

- What's a caregiver to do? First, work with the physician of the person with Alzheimer's to stabilize his sleeping patterns. After eliminating other possible causes of insomnia (lack of exercise, continence problems, etc.), a mild prescription sleep aid may be the safest, best course of action. Next, see your own physician if you are still having trouble sleeping. It's too important not to get to the bottom of it.

- No matter your situation, know that you can find a solution to your sleep troubles. Don't give up until you do.

CARPE DIEM

If you haven't been getting enough sleep, make an appointment with your primary care physician today.

28.

QUIET YOUR MIND

- Is your mind racing? Jumping from thought to thought? Does it feel full and overwhelmed by your situation? Buddhists call this churning mental chaos "papanca," which means monkey mind. This stressful jumping from thought to thought can resemble a monkey jumping from limb to limb in a tree.

- Your body's natural relaxation response can help to quiet this monkey mind. There are many ways, but one basic technique it to "clear your mind." With daily practice it can help you feel refreshed and more energetic.

- Here is one way to do this:

  - Find a quiet spot that will allow your mind to feel at peace. Sit still, loosen any tight clothing, kick off your shoes, relax your body into a comfortable position, and off you go.
  - Close your eyes and begin slow breathing. Monitor your deep breaths with a hand on your stomach.
  - Mentally focus on a peaceful world with a thought or image, like a mountain stream or a quiet beach. If other thoughts creep in, just relax, breathe deeply, and try again. Spend at least several minutes with your mind focused on this peaceful sensation.
  - Stretch and exhale deeply to complete the exercise.

CARPE DIEM

In your busy world, especially if you are a caregiver, finding time to enjoy quiet and uninterrupted peace and solace is difficult. But you can make the conscious decision to relax and clear your mind by setting aside 5 to 10 minutes daily to practice this quieting exercise.

29.

CREATE ROOM FOR HOPE

- As the person's illness progresses and she changes, you may experience a loss of a companion and a relationship important to you. You may grieve for the "way she used to be." You will likely feel sad or discouraged.

- When you are grieving, sometimes even little things can make you feel sad or cry. You may feel that tearfulness or sadness is welling up inside you. These sad feelings may be mixed with depression or fatigue. They may come and go, but they are a normal part of the experience of grief and the need to mourn.

- Unfortunately, with a chronic illness, grief can go on and on. Families often find it increasingly sad to watch the suffering of a loved one as his disease progresses.

- Your sadness may not be understood by others, especially if the person who is ill still appears well. People may tell you, "Be grateful you still have your husband" or "Keep a stiff upper lip." You may feel you should keep your feelings of sadness to yourself. Resist this urge. Let your sadness out. Cry when you feel like. Let your close family and friends know how you feel. Letting your sadness out will create room for hope.

CARPE DIEM

Picture yourself in a closed, stuffy room with the blinds drawn. You are unhappy in this room. Now open the blinds, open the windows and open the door. Notice that when you let the bad air out, fresh air also rushes in.

30.

LET YOUR TEARS FLOW

"Tears of sorrow, grief, and desperation can turn inward. Tears of determination, hope, and compassion can be turned outward. Healing tears move to action, can bring growth."

– Author Unknown

• To mourn means to let your inner emotions out. Crying allows your sadness to leave your body by flowing out with your tears. Crying is a release. It is letting down your guard to be fully there, in the moment, with your sadness. After crying, people often feel calmer and more settled.

• Tears are the body's way of expressing sadness, anxiety, fear, and a host of other emotions.

• You may find yourself crying at unexpected times or places. We call these episodes "griefbursts," and they are a natural part of the grief experience. Griefbursts make some people uncomfortable, since many of us do not know how to be present to others in pain. Try to find someone who can support you and sit with you while you cry.

• Remember: Not everyone cries during times of loss, and if you are not feeling the need to cry, this doesn't mean there is something wrong with you. If you are not a crier, release feelings of sadness by spending time outdoors, writing, or talking with others.

CARPE DIEM

Sometimes a good cry can bring a real sense of release and relief. Write down how you are feeling to bring your emotions to the surface, then, if you feel like it, release them through crying. Or simply be open to crying when you feel like crying.

31.

EXPRESS ANGER IN HEALTHY WAYS

• Anger or feelings of protest often come up when we experience personal crises. Anger is a completely normal human emotion. But when it gets out of control, it can cause problems in all aspects of our lives, including work, relationships, and our own sense of contentment.

• Anger can mask other emotions such as fear, frustration, resentment, or even feeling disrespected. Instead of experiencing these emotions, you feel anger instead. Your true emotions are disguised. Your feelings may be complex about your loved one's Alzheimer's, but they may sometimes come to the surface as anger.

• There are a few ways to deal with anger when it arises. One is to express it. Anger that is expressed assertively—not aggressively—brings relief and helps us get our needs met. But expressing it too assertively, especially around someone with Alzheimer's, can escalate his behavior and makes things worse. A good way to calm down in the presence of someone with Alzheimer's is to distract him from the behavior or situation that is upsetting you. Or walk away, taking a mental break and slowing your breathing and heartbeat.

• Anger that is held inside can cause heart disease, stroke, depression, and substance abuse. It can also leave you feeling cynical and hostile to others, even your loved one. Take steps to actively express and resolve your feelings of bitterness, anger, and resentment as you mourn your losses.

CARPE DIEM

Actively express your anger by venting to a friend or family
member, writing down your feelings, giving it form and
shape in art, or exercising. Or calm yourself if you need to
by taking time alone for a walk in the park or meditating. If
you need extra help understanding and expressing your anger,
consider making an appointment with a counselor.

32.

MAKE PEACE WITH GUILT

- Throughout the grieving process, guilt is a common—though not universal—feeling among those who love someone with Alzheimer's.

- If you feel guilty (and you may not), your feelings may be related to:

  - thinking you could have done something differently, or regretting things in the relationship.
  - being able to enjoy life when your loved one may not.
  - wondering if you somehow played a role in contributing to the disease.
  - having negative thoughts about the person with the disease— or wishing that his suffering would come to an end.
  - having conflicts with family members because they are uninvolved or critical of the care being provided.
  - placing unrealistic expectations on yourself and thinking, "I must be perfect" or "I must do everything."
  - feeling you have failed if you can't be part of the day-to-day caregiving or are no longer able to take care of your loved one at home.

- Accept that you do not have control over this disease. You are doing the best you can. Any feelings of guilt you may have are natural and understandable, but they are a symptom of underlying feelings of helplessness. We do not like to feel helpless.

- If you are feeling guilty, find ways to express these feelings. Talk to an empathetic friend or neighbor.

CARPE DIEM

Make a list of the things that you are feeling guilty about.
Light a candle for each of these guilts. Now, say out loud that
you forgive yourself for each of them as you blow out the
candles. Feel the peace of self-awareness and forgiveness.

33.

CONFRONT YOUR FEARS

- Fear is a distressing but normal emotion we experience when we feel threatened.

- The problem with fear is that it comes from the amygdala—a prehistoric part of our brain whose job it is to sense danger and keep us alive.

- The fears you may be experiencing right now, however, are probably not due to imminent threats on your life. They are longer-term, quality-of-life fears. What will the person I love be like next year? Five years from now? Who will take care of him? How will healthcare costs be covered? What will I do without him? What if I get Alzheimer's?

- These kinds of fears naturally eat away at us, but the secret is that they can be quieted if not silenced altogether by looking them full in the face. Express them. Talk to others about them. Seek out information and make plans. Then try to let go of anything that's left, anything you can't control.

CARPE DIEM

What are you most afraid of right now? Today, talk to someone about this fear and notice how you feel after you've voiced it.

34.

DEVELOP A NEW SELF-IDENTITY

- As mourners, we have a number of needs that must be met if we are to go on to heal and live and love deeply again. One of these needs is to develop a new self-identity.

- Part of your self-identity comes from the relationships you have with other people. When someone with whom you have a relationship is diagnosed with dementia or Alzheimer's, your self-identity, or the way you see yourself, naturally begins to change. Your role in the relationship may be in flux. You may go from being a spouse or a child to a parent-like caregiver. You will need to mourn the old you as well as the old him.

- The disease may be requiring you to take on new roles that had been filled by the person who is ill. After all, someone still has to take out the garbage, someone still has to buy the groceries, someone still has to balance the checkbook. You confront your changed identity every time you do something that used to be done by the person who is ill. This can be very hard work and, at times, can leave you feeling very drained of emotional, physical, and spiritual energy.

- Many people discover that as they work on this need, they ultimately discover some positive aspects of their changed self-identities. You may develop a renewed confidence in yourself, for example. You may develop a more caring, kind, and sensitive part of yourself. You may develop an assertive part of your identity that empowers you to go on living even though you continue to feel a sense of loss.

CARPE DIEM

Do you have a Facebook page? Maybe now is the time to make one. After all, your Facebook page is your "this is me!" proclamation to the world. Practically speaking, Facebook may also help you reconnect with others you've lost track of and express your feelings about Alzheimer's disease.

35.

MAKE FRIENDS WITH FEELINGS OF RELIEF

- It is normal to experience bursts of relief now and then during your grief journey. Feelings of relief mean that your heart senses a burden being lifted.

- If the person with Alzheimer's stops exhibiting a troublesome symptom or behavior, you may feel relieved. If you are the primary caregiver and someone provides you with respite care or you decide it is time for the person to live in a long-term care facility, you may feel relieved. When the person with Alzheimer's dies, you may feel relief mixed with sadness and other emotions.

- Of course, many times feelings of relief are followed by feelings of guilt. We often feel guilty when what is good for us is less than ideal for someone else.

- Just remember that relief is a blessing. It de-stresses and cleanses. It is a sign of anxiety lifted. Allow yourself to revel in the lightness.

CARPE DIEM

When you are feeling relief, you may be in a frame of mind to feel grateful, too. Today, write a note of thanks to someone you feel grateful for.

36.

FIND PEOPLE WHO GIVE ENCOURAGEMENT

"Who helps me in a hardship truly is my friend."

— Swahili proverb

• Loving someone with Alzheimer's is often discouraging. It can be devastating to watch a loved one regress. Having others who support and encourage you can make all the difference in keeping your spirits up.

• We have noticed that when we are struggling with a challenge in life, our friends and family members tend to fall into the "law of thirds." About a third of people you know will be supportive and encouraging; about a third will be neutral (not much help but at least not negative); and a third will be openly discouraging and sometimes harmful.

• With the discouragement you have felt from dealing with the effects of dementia, it is important for you to seek out people who will offer you encouragement in your life and support you—not shame, belittle, or discourage you.

• If no one in the "helpful third" comes to mind, call your local Alzheimer's Association to get in touch with supportive people.

CARPE DIEM

In Biblical times, Barnabas, whose name means "son of encouragement," earned his nickname by encouraging his friends, even when others gave up on them. Make a list of the Barnabases in your life. Reach out and spend time with those people. Allow their gift of encouragement to support you in your journey through the losses of Alzheimer's.

37.

ASK WHY

- Major life transitions, like the diagnosis of Alzheimer's in a loved one, may leave you wondering about the meaning and purpose of life. With the loss of normalcy in your life, you may feel dumbfounded and have the desire to ask why.

- "Why?" questions can come on uncontrollably and often precede "How?" questions. "Why did this happen?" often comes before "How will I survive this?" It is normal to ask questions like:

  - Why this, why now?
  - Why the person I love, why me?
  - Why did it have to happen this way?
  - Why am I here, dealing with this disease?
  - Why do good things have to come to an end?

- The answers will come from within. But you may decide there are no answers to some of these questions. This disease may never make complete sense to you.

CARPE DIEM

Write down a list of the "Why?" questions you have about your loved one's illness. Explore these with someone you trust—someone who will allow you to ask without feeling a need to answer.

38.

REMEMBER THE GOOD TIMES

- Alzheimer's tends to affect long-term memory less than shorter-term memory. A person with the disease may not be able to remember what he did this morning, but he may have clear memories from 20 or more years ago. He may even seem to believe that he is living in this earlier time.

- Take advantage of this time warp to recollect and re-experience the good times that you enjoyed together. That terrific vacation you shared. The fun experiences within the family. The laughter and animation at get-togethers. It may still be there for you to share with the person you love.

- Not only is remembering the good times a welcome experience for your loved one, it will do you good as well. Healthy mourning of your losses involves reviewing, remembering, and realistically re-experiencing the associated feelings you have had. Remember the fun, and plan to have more in the future.

CARPE DIEM

Take time today to think about the most fun times you ever spent with the person with Alzheimer's. If you can, talk about those times with him and see what memories he has of the event. If the person with Alzheimer's is not nearby or can no longer carry on a conversation with you, consider writing your memories down in the form of a letter: Dear _____, I remember when…." Share the letter with someone else who cares about the person with Alzheimer's.

39.

KEEP A JOURNAL

- Writing can be a healing process. As psychologist James Pennebaker explains, "Not only is the pen mightier than the sword, it is mightier than the armies of anxieties that keep us captive to stress."

- Writing about your losses can help you openly and actively mourn. Putting your experiences on paper helps you to:

  - give voice to your emotions.
  - process your feelings.
  - create a meaningful story about your experiences with the disease.
  - release your tension through words.
  - sort through the "hows" and "whys" of the losses of Alzheimer's.
  - feel a sense of control.
  - see progress in your journey.

- Keep a daily journal on a notebook or your computer. List not only the events of the day but also your feelings.

CARPE DIEM

If you are not sure how to get started, try a "writing web." On a piece of paper make a circle. Write down a main thought in the circle. Maybe it is "Alzheimer's losses" or "miss my friends" or particular feelings such as "sadness" or "loneliness." Now draw a line to another circle and write down the first thing that comes into your head. If you have new thoughts related to this, draw more lines and circles. Or you can go back to the main circle and start again with a new idea. Don't worry about spelling or punctuation; just let your ideas flow. If you fill one side of the paper turn it over and keep going.

40.

LET WATER REFRESH YOUR SOUL

- Most people appreciate the natural healing powers of water. It symbolizes refreshment and replenishment. Your life and soul may feel dry and barren from the stresses of dealing with this disease. Your inner self may need refreshment.

- When you spend time around water, you embrace its tranquility and flow. Your life may lack this sense of peace and smoothness right now. Experiencing flowing water can reawaken this within you.

- Consider one of these experiences:
    - Visit the ocean and watch, listen to, and feel its ebb and flow.
    - Take a hike and sit by a mountain stream or waterfall.
    - Sit by a pond or lake.
    - Take a long shower or sit in a hot tub.
    - Float in a pool or lake.
    - Walk in the rain.
    - Fill a kid's pool with water in your backyard and sit in it.

- Water is one of the four basic elements of the world, a provider of life. It is pure and precious and brings healing when we experience it. Breaking water, like waves, can release negative ions. Negative ions have been shown to purify the air and increase your energy levels. Take a break today and spend time near the healing presence of water. Refresh your inner soul.

CARPE DIEM

Take one of these examples of a water experience, or think of one on your own, and set a date within the next few days to experience the healing power of water.

41.

BE ARTFUL IN GRIEF

- Many people find that making art is a meaningful way to express their grief.

- Even if you've never considered yourself "artistic," you can still create. And creation is a powerful antidote to feelings of depression, powerlessness, and despair.

- Sketch. Finger paint. Sign up for a pottery class. Knit. Scrapbook.

- Consider getting your loved one involved in the Alzheimer's Memories in the Making art program. Share making art together.

- Of course, the visual arts are just one form of art. Play an instrument. Write a song. Try out for a role in a community theater production. Sing in a choir.

- Whether you know it or not, whether you believe it or not, you have art inside of you. Unleash it.

CARPE DIEM

Today, take photos of the person with Alzheimer's. Be creative.
Try to capture the things you still love best about her—her
hands, her smile, the tilt of her head. Whatever remains that
you can connect with, capture it while you still can.

42.

MAKE USE OF RITUAL

- When words are inadequate, ceremony speaks volumes.

- Ceremony assists in reality, recall, support, expression, transcendence.

- You might find it helpful right now to participate in ritualistic practices such as attending worship services, daily prayer, yoga, or walking a labyrinth. Even participating in an Alzheimer's Walk is making using of the power of ritual.

- Our culture doesn't always understand the value of ceremony. Don't expect that everyone around you will understand your desire to make use of ritual. However, don't allow their lack of understanding to persuade you to forego ceremonies both now and later, including planning a meaningful funeral.

CARPE DIEM

Hold a tree planting in honor of the person with Alzheimer's. Invite friends over and ask everyone to pitch in. When the tree is planted, say a few words about what the person with Alzheimer's means to you and how you look forward to this tree carrying on his legacy in the decades to come.

43.

SEEK THE SPIRITUAL

- Your mind, body, and spirit are interconnected. When you neglect one part of your being, the other parts of yourself are affected. Your spiritual needs are often harder to recognize than physical or emotional needs.

- The stress and grief of dealing with Alzheimer's may have brought you to a spiritual crisis. You may be asking questions like: "Why did this have to happen?" or "Why would God allow something like Alzheimer's to exist?" You may be re-examining your values or even re-evaluating your purpose and meaning in life.

- Some activities that may help meet your spiritual needs have a basis in religion, like prayer, talking with clergy, prayer groups, Bible study, or attending religious services. Other spiritual activities outside of religion may also help, such as support groups, walks in nature, contemplative practices like yoga or tai chi, or mindfulness, which is paying attention to what you are thinking and feeling in the moment.

- Take the time to allow your spirit to come forward in a spiritual practice that works for you.

CARPE DIEM

Take a few minutes today to express your spirituality. What spiritual needs do you feel? Give these needs a voice and allow your spirit to step forward by engaging in a contemplative practice like prayer, yoga, tai chi—or find one of your own.

44.

CREATE A SANCTUARY

- A sanctuary is a place of refuge and safety. It's somewhere removed from the overwhelming problems and chaos of the day. It's a place that allows your mind to unwind and find peace. It's a place that allows your body to loosen and relax. With the stress of grieving and taking care of the changes wrought by Alzheimer's, you may need to create such a sanctuary to help renew yourself.

- You can turn a room or just a corner of the room into a cozy spot that reminds you to relax and enjoy. Pick a spot that is quiet but inviting. Have a comfortable place to sit and something pleasant to look at or listen to, like a small water feature. Consider incense or some other fragrance.

- Decorate your space with photos or art that you enjoy. Keep a supply of your favorite chocolate, nuts, or low-fat snacks nearby, along with books, music, and a journal or sketchpad. You decide; it's your place.

- Now be sure to schedule your day so that you can regularly spend some time in your sanctuary, away from the hustle and bustle of your life.

CARPE DIEM

Take a moment and think about where in your house you could create a sanctuary. What would you like to have in it? How can you schedule some regular time there? Take the steps to make your sanctuary a reality.

45.

RETREAT TO STILLNESS

- Sitting in stillness with your grief will honor your deeper voice of quiet wisdom. Create regular opportunities for moments of stillness and reflection in your life.

- You may need to get out of the routine of your busy life to find stillness. Go to the park to sit under a tree, or take a hike in a wooded area. Sit on your porch with a glass of iced tea, or go to a hilltop to look at the vista. Or it may be as simple as taking a bubble bath or sitting by the fireplace and watching the embers. Find what works for you.

- However you do it, creating stillness is good for your spirit. Without stillness, our bodies, minds, and spirits have no place for rest and rejuvenation. If we do not calm ourselves at a deeper level, we feel disconnected, rushed, uncertain, and overwhelmed.

- Especially if you are the primary caregiver, you may feel you have too many things to do in dealing with this terrible disease. There appears to be no time for stillness.

- But stillness can be a path through the chaos. The quietness of sitting in stillness can allow your soul to ever so slowly be restored. With stillness you can learn contentment and peace.

CARPE DIEM

Take a moment right now to sit in a quiet place. Close your eyes, take a deep breath and slowly exhale. Experience the stillness around you. Hear the distant noises and notice the faint light you see through your eyelids. Lean back and relax into the quietness.

46.

EMBRACE THE LIGHT OF NATURE

- Experiencing the beauty of nature is a naturally healing experience. When our inner thoughts and emotional experiences are dark, the light of a spectacular panorama or even the quiet beauty of a flower can help us move from the darkness to light.

- Nature can remind us that there is still peace, harmony, and wonderful things to experience within our world. We can let the peace and harmony of nature replenish our spirits.

- Sunlight itself is a powerful healer. It replenishes the vitamin D within our body to help improve our energy levels. It can work on our internal clocks to allow the natural release of melatonin, which enhances sleep. Regular doses of sunlight can keep us from falling into depression and seasonal affective disorder (SAD) in the winter.

- Not far from your home are amazing streams, rivers, parks, and recreational areas. Hiking trails, forests, and bike paths await you. Take the time to embrace the healing light of nature.

CARPE DIEM

Take a walk in a natural area. Sit and experience the wondrous light of nature. See the beauty of trees and water. Feel the caress of the breeze. Hear the sounds of birds and wildlife. Let the peaceful light of nature enter your soul.

47.

MOURN AT YOUR CROSSROADS

- The Kongo people of Africa, whose religion is a mixture of native African and Christian beliefs, use a symbol of a cross within a circle to represent the crossroads of the spiritual, which means the physical boundary where living people, their ancestors, and the spiritual meet.

- Other boundaries, such as the horizon where the earth touches the sky, are also thought to be junctions where the material and the spiritual meet, as are:

  - where water and land meet
  - where the river meets the riverbank
  - where the beach and ocean collide
  - where the mountain touches the clouds

- It may take effort to reach one of these naturally spiritual places, but if you do, there is a good chance it will relax your body, bring calmness to your mind, and open your spirit to peace. When you reach a crossroads, breathe deep, walk, pray, write, meditate, do whatever it is that permits you to be present to the moment. Allow the grief that you feel to join you and express itself.

CARPE DIEM

Do you remember experiencing spiritual feelings at crossroads in your past? Where was it? At the beach? On a mountain? Relive the memory, or better yet go to one of these places.

Join your loved one's new world

The person with Alzheimer's disease is living in a new and ever-changing reality. He can no longer fully live in your world…but you can take steps to live in his. By being present to his in-the-now feelings, needs, and abilities, you may still be able to share moments of joy and love.

48.

JOIN YOUR LOVED ONE

- Don't look at people with Alzheimer's and just write them off. Look your loved one in the eye, and talk to him directly. Join him where he is.

- Don't panic or take it personally if your loved one makes mistakes, because he will. He will repeat himself, he will misplace things, and he will get lost. He will forget your name and what you said just a few minutes ago. But, he will also try hard to compensate for his cognitive losses. Join him in this effort.

- To allow him to function as fully as possible, empower him, and avoid limiting him. Work with him to develop tools to function around the losses in memory, language, and cognition.

- Encourage his involvement in support groups, and you join one too. We can help each other, both people with dementia and their caregivers and friends, to navigate the maze of Alzheimer's. We must live for each day. Just because your loved may forget it tomorrow doesn't mean he didn't live each second today. Just because he may forget today, doesn't mean today didn't matter.

CARPE DIEM

Take a few minutes and write down on paper ways you can join your loved one. Consider ways to communicate, ways to empower him, and ways to help him compensate for his losses, among others.

49.

MEET HER WHERE SHE IS

"Never question, chastise, or try to reason with the (Alzheimer's) patient. Join him in his current 'place' or time, no matter when or where that may be, and find joy with him there."

– Joanne Koenig Coste

- Since your loved one may not be able to communicate in words what may seem to be simple information, you will need to join her world to understand what she is experiencing and to communicate your love.

- When you are in the presence of the person with Alzheimer's, try to create moments of success, avoid moments of failure, and praise frequently and with sincerity. Find and share joy whenever possible.

- When you are not near the person with Alzheimer's but would still like to express your thoughts and feelings, consider sending small tokens of your love. Mail a postcard, order a favorite candy, or frame and send a special photo.

- It's common for those who love someone with Alzheimer's to distance themselves as much as possible because "nothing is getting through." Yet those among you who provide around-the-clock care to someone with Alzheimer's know that moments of awareness and connection sometimes surface when you least expect them. And even when they don't, expressing your own thoughts and feelings has intrinsic value.

CARPE DIEM

Do something to connect with the person you love or express your thoughts and feelings to her today.

50.

TRY TO UNDERSTAND WHAT ALZHEIMER'S MIGHT FEEL LIKE

"Sometimes something is familiar to me. Most times there is no recognition of the fabric of my life. Only frayed remnants of who I once was."

– Joanne Koenig Coste

- Many people talk about what Alzheimer's looks like, including doctors, family members and friends. But think to yourself: What does the person with Alzheimer's experience?

- Early on, most people with the disease do recognize changes in themselves, but they often attribute them to stress or other causes. Sometimes they admit to knowing something is wrong but seem unconcerned with figuring out what the problem is. Sadly, this lack of self-awareness goes hand in hand with the apathy and indifference that Alzheimer's can cause.

- On the other hand, many people with Alzheimer's do know something is wrong with their behavior and thinking. They are often perplexed, unsure, or uneasy about their memory loss. This uncertainty can engulf them.

- People with Alzheimer's are often afraid of making mistakes and may only be intermittently aware of their memory loss. They may feel "I'm not myself." Some people describe losing their spark, their zest for life. The world they live in is frightening, and they are fuzzy and foggy about what is happening. In essence, they have become lost in the corridors of their mind.

CARPE DIEM

Today, take five or ten minutes to try to imagine how you would feel if you had Alzheimer's. Feel the fear of not knowing if you are doing things correctly. The frustration of not being able to remember familiar things. The uncertainty of what is happening to you. Now see if you can detect some of these feelings in your loved one.

51.

GET INTO THE WORLD
OF THE SENSES

- Alzheimer's takes people out of the world of words, logic, and reason and brings them into the landscape of feeling and sensing. To communicate you may need to provide outlets that allow the person you care about to express herself through her senses, and to understand you may need to join her in this world.

- Appeal to your loved one's senses through art, massage, the pleasant scent of food cooking, warmth, hugs, and, maybe best of all, music. Music can be great for calming, motivating, and just having fun.

- When you are feeling your grief, try different sensory techniques for exploring it and expressing it. Evocative smells can stir memories and transport us to a different time and place. Try some essential oils. Petting a dog or stroking a cat helps soothe frayed nerves. Eating chocolate releases endorphins, which can counteract sadness. Play music that matches your mood.

CARPE DIEM

Most of us rely primarily on our sense of sight for taking in the world. Today, make a point of indulging one of your other senses in some way. Try calling on your sense of smell or touch to help you express whatever thoughts and feelings inside you are most urgent right now.

52.

RELY ON BODY LANGUAGE

- Words are only one part of communication. Even when words fail, people with Alzheimer's can still retain other modes of understanding and being understood. They may well get meaning from your body language and facial expressions, and you may be able to read their emotions as well.

- Try paying attention to the person's eyes and determining meaning through voice tone and gestures. It's like still being able to understand the plot of a movie, even with the sound turned off.

- We all use gestures, pictures, voice tone and pitch, facial expressions, and body movements to communicate with friends, family, and even strangers. Body language can be even more honest and reliable, at times, than words.

- Try using body language as one way of expressing your own grief. Hug the people you care about, including the person who has Alzheimer's. Gesture your anger. Curl up in a ball when you feel sad. Let your body be your instrument when your thoughts and feelings are too profound for words.

CARPE DIEM

Right now, close your eyes and assess how you are feeling, emotionally and spiritually. Move your body in a way that expresses those feelings.

53.

FIND A GOOD PLACE TO TALK

- When you are talking with someone who has a hard time communicating, it's important to choose a good place to talk. The best place, first of all, is a quiet place.

- It is hard to understand speech when there is a lot of noise. This is especially true for people with Alzheimer's, since they are easily distracted and can struggle in a noisy room. So, turn down the music, shut off the television, stop the dishwasher, and avoid other household noises when talking to your loved one.

- Peaceful surroundings will help a person's understanding. If you remove distractions, like playful pets, he may be able to focus on the talk at hand. Create a smaller, more intimate space for conversation with a room divider, folding door, curtain hung from the ceiling, folding screen, or privacy wall.

- Keep the group small. People with dementia communicate best when face-to-face with one other person. Have only one conversation at a time.

- Of course, all of this holds true for you and your need for focused, intimate conversation as you share the story of your loss and grief, as well.

CARPE DIEM

Arrange to have a conversation with someone in a quiet, peaceful, intimate place today. Notice what a difference it makes for you.

54.

VALIDATE FEELINGS

- For the person with Alzheimer's, communication problems may begin at the same time as other thought process problems, which makes the situation even more difficult. The slow loss of coherent speech is complicated by the declining ability to draw conclusions.

- Difficulty with language can cause emotional outbursts. Imagine the anguish of having your ability to talk to the people you love, chat with friends, and even greet strangers slowly taken away.

- Remember it is the emotion behind the person's failing words that is important. It is the emotions that need to be validated.

- Likewise, your feelings need to be honored. The person with Alzheimer's may no longer be capable of validating your feelings, but others are. Talk to your friends and family members who have good listening ears. People sometimes say that talk won't change anything, but this is far from true. Expressing your thoughts and feelings to others is an essential form of mourning, and mourning is the path to your eventual healing.

CARPE DIEM

Has the person with Alzheimer's had an emotional outburst during a recent conversation? What do you think he was feeling? If this happens again, try validating the feelings behind the outburst: "I think you must be feeling worried but are having trouble saying the words. Are you worried?"

55.

FIND WAYS TO EMPOWER

- To preserve dignity, look for ways to help the person with Alzheimer's compensate, cope, and adapt to her ever-changing life. Remember that the ability to self-reflect will continue despite the disease. Finding ways to empower her to continue to feel productive and of value must be part of your new mindset.

- Some ways you might try to communicate empowerment and connection include:

    - Finding old photos and sitting down to look them over with your loved one. Ask him what he remembers about the photo. This often triggers long-term memories.
    - Playing simple games like identifying things around the house to stimulate language skills.
    - Thinking about activities your loved one used to enjoy and finding ways for her to still participate in or even watch these activities, such as painting, taking photos, playing the piano, gardening or other hobbies.
    - Calling on the phone regularly or scheduling a time to take regular walks to a local restaurant for exercise as well as social time.
    - Playing games or dancing to stimulate movement.
    - Playing music, continuing to decorate the house for the holidays, or simply setting a nice table to provide a stimulating environment that appeals to the senses.

- Of course, empowering yourself to fully live your own life and mourn your many losses is just as important. If you are a caregiver, this may mean being proactive in finding caregiving help.

CARPE DIEM

Make a list of the activities that may help empower the person you love. Then make a list of activities that would help empower you.

56.

STAY CLOSE

- For the person you love, being diagnosed with Alzheimer's may feel like being branded with a scarlet "A." She is now someone with dementia. She may begin to define herself by her disease, which is disheartening because Alzheimer's is progressive and incurable.

- But a person is always and ultimately more than his disease. He is more than what he does and more than what he remembers. As humans we are all fundamentally more than all of this.

- Always remember that the person you care about is not just an Alzheimer's patient. She may be a wife, a mother, a friend, a grandmother. Whoever she is, she is still worthy of love and joy in those relationships. Help her retain the love and joy by remaining close to her.

- It's up to you. Her brain may no longer work well, but she has ears for unconditional listening, shoulders for crying on, and arms for hugging. Especially if you don't live nearby, it may be tempting to stop visiting, especially if the person no longer seems to know you. But we believe (and have experienced ourselves) that love expressed is always love received. Love unexpressed, on the other hand, is future regret in the making.

CARPE DIEM

To feel close to your loved one, it may help to read books from the perspective of an Alzheimer's patient. Try *Still Alice* by Lisa Genova or *Turn of Mind* by Alice LaPlante. Or just spend more time with your loved one and be present to her mood, her needs, and her feelings.

57.

UNDERSTAND WHY PEOPLE WITH ALZHEIMER'S DO WHAT THEY DO

"You can't regret what you can't remember."

– Lisa Birnbach

- The brain is a very complex and mysterious organ. The very nature of brain injuries can make them difficult to live with. Injury to the brain can cause alterations in thoughts, emotions, personality, and the ability to reason. Many of the changes seen in Alzheimer's arise from structural and chemical changes in the brain.

- Most illnesses that cause dementia develop gradually, unlike head trauma or stroke, in which changes are more sudden. Consequently, the behavior changes can be puzzling because they gradually occur in a person who often looks well.

- Different parts of the brain perform different tasks. In dementia, damage is done to many areas of the brain, so there can be an uneven distribution of emotional and behavioral changes. When brain damage is uneven, the person may do things that don't make sense to us.

- You may wonder which behaviors are caused by the disease and which are deliberate and willful. Try to separate the brain disease from the soul you love. When people with Alzheimer's say or do things that don't make sense or seem nasty or deliberate, the disease is almost always to blame.

- When things get tough, remember that the person you are caring for is often miserable, too, and is doing the best that he can.

CARPE DIEM

Picture the person with Alzheimer's as he was as a child. You might even use a photo from his childhood for this visualization. Now imagine holding this child on your lap and kissing his cheek. You love and forgive him. Remember, this child is the same person, the same soul, who has Alzheimer's today.

58.

UNDERSTAND BEING LOST IN TIME

- With Alzheimer's, one loses the ability to judge the passage of time. Your loved one may repeatedly ask you what time it is, thinking hours have passed when it has been only a few minutes.

- Besides this defect of memory, it appears that dementia can also affect the internal clock that keeps our regular schedule of sleeping, waking, and eating. Recognize that this irregularity of sleeping and waking, though irritating, is not intentional. It is the result of the loss of brain function.

- The ability to read a clock may be lost early in the disease, and not being able to keep track of time can worry the forgetful person. She may not even know what she is worried about, but there may be a general sense of anxiety, which in turn makes her ask what time it is.

- Sometimes a person with Alzheimer's feels that you have deserted him when you have been gone only briefly. Be patient with him and comfort him, for he is lost in time.

CARPE DIEM

If the person you love is struggling with his loss of the sense of time, try one of these ideas: Set a timer or an old-fashioned hourglass so he will hear or see when time has passed. Consider writing a note to let him know you will be back at a certain time. He may be more patient as long as you have left a clue that he can comprehend.

59.

CREATE A PEACEFUL ENVIRONMENT

- A peaceful environment is much easier to function in for a person with Alzheimer's. If you are a caregiver, consider keeping background sounds, like those from television, stereos, and radios, at a low level. Try eliminating clutter and simplifying the person's surroundings.

- The hearing of a person with Alzheimer's does not typically change. But as her brain changes, her interpretation of sound changes over time. Research shows that many of the sounds we take for granted can actually disturb people with progressive dementia.

- As a mourner, you too might benefit from a review of your environment. What in your home or daily workspace (or even your car) causes you to feel anxious or annoyed? Noise-cancelling headphones can do wonders to eliminate unavoidable sounds that you find irritating. Cleaning and de-cluttering shelves, cabinets, and surfaces often helps people feel more organized and serene. Painting walls a soothing or neutral color, such as a pale blue or a beigey-brown, may also make a big difference.

- You probably know someone who would be happy to help you tackle a cleaning and organizing project. Friends and family members often want to help but don't know how. If presented with a specific request, however, they will often tackle it with relish. All you have to do is ask.

CARPE DIEM

Take a look at your environment. Take one
step today to make it more peaceful.

60.

KEEP A ONE-DAY-AT-A-TIME CALENDAR

"There's only us. There's only this. Forget regret, or life is yours to miss. No other road. No other way. No day but today."

— From the musical *Rent*

- Living one day at a time may be the most difficult challenge to set before modern man, yet it is *your* challenge.

- Your grief will change from week to week and month to month, but today you can acknowledge it for what it is and you can choose to express it.

- If you are a caregiver to the person with Alzheimer's, you know that every day is different and it's impossible to predict what will happen tomorrow. Therefore you must live in the present. If there is a gift of Alzheimer's, perhaps this is it.

- Living in the present is fatiguing. Most of us are used to distracting ourselves with the future. To counteract the fatigue, plan several treats for yourself throughout each day. Call a friend. Watch your favorite sit-com. Indulge in a cookie. Take a cat-nap.

CARPE DIEM

Buy a small desk calendar that displays one day at a time. Place it somewhere you'll see if often. Use it as a visual reminder that you are living this day and only this day.

61.

PRACTICE PATIENCE—WITH YOUR LOVED ONE AND YOURSELF

"Lord, teach me to be patient with life, with people, with myself. I try to speed things along too much, and I push for results before the time is right. Teach me to trust your sense of timing. Teach me to slow down enough to appreciate life."

— Patience Prayer

- We are an impatient society. The digital age has taught us to expect results immediately. Instant messaging, digital photos, fast food, downloadable books—sometimes it seems everything we want and need is available not just quickly but instantaneously, and we expect it.

- Alzheimer's, however, is rarely a fast disease. It may well be a part of your life for many years. So, when you are grieving the slow loss of someone you love to Alzheimer's disease, learning to practice patience may well be the key to your survival and eventual healing.

- Be patient with the person with Alzheimer's, with your family, with caregivers, and with yourself. At its core, patience really means being nonjudgmental, moment by moment. Each moment that you live, you can choose whether to judge the moment as good or bad or to accept it as it is and respond with love.

- "I feel sad," your body might tell you. "Yes, I acknowledge your sadness," you reply. "I will witness your sadness as long as you need."

- Patience in the moment is essential, but patience in the long-term—what we also call endurance—is equally important. Look back and see how far you have already come on this journey through Alzheimer's. Have you found any satisfaction and joy on the journey?

CARPE DIEM

Try practicing patience in your next conversation with your loved one. Try not to finish her sentences, rush her ideas, or pressure her responses. You have as much time as you need to communicate. Take the time.

62.

DEAR FAMILY, GET IT TOGETHER

- Families have a choice in deciding how to care for someone with Alzheimer's: they can be helpful and supportive to one another, or they can create roadblocks and bad feelings.

- Rivalry among family members can surface when it is time to make important decisions. This can destroy any will to compromise. Now is not the time to share how you really feel about your relatives or remind them of their shortcomings. If you want people to reach agreement, skip the accusations.

- Even if families get along well, they may simply disagree on what is best for the person with Alzheimer's. Family members may listen to a well-meaning friend or a doctor who says the person's problems are just a normal part of aging. This can obstruct the necessary interventions that need to be made.

- Families can also disagree about finances. They may not be able to afford the high cost of medical care, may not know where to turn, and may not have access to less expensive options. This can create worry and conflict.

- Social workers generally say the first step in moving a family forward is finding something that you can agree on, no matter how simple. This can start everyone moving towards compromise and consensus. If possible, include the person with Alzheimer's in the conversation and start moving forward together.

CARPE DIEM

What do you and your family members agree on regarding your loved one's care? Where do you disagree? List both. At your next family meeting, first discuss areas where you agree. Then move to areas where you don't. Can you find ways for compromise and consensus? Remember to get mad at the disease—not each other.

63.

IF YOU ARE A CAREGIVER, GO WITH THE FLOW

"There is no substitute for the love of an Alzheimer's caregiver."

– Bob DeMarco

- Be informed. The more you know about Alzheimer's, the more effective you will be in devising strategies to manage the behavioral symptoms, even if you are not the main caregiver.

- Share your concerns with the person with Alzheimer's. When a person is only mildly to moderately impaired, he can still take part in managing the problem. You may be able to share with each other your grief and worries, and together you can devise memory strategies. Mildly impaired people may benefit from counseling to help them accept and adjust to their limitations.

- Try to solve the most frustrating problems one at a time. Often day-to-day problems seem the most insurmountable. Getting her to take her bath, getting her dressed, or getting supper prepared and put away can become a daily ordeal. If you are feeling like you're at the end of your rope, single out one thing that you can change to make life easier and work on that.

- Use your common sense and imagination. Adaptation is the key. If you are struggling with getting something done or changed, ask if it needs to be done at all. If a person insists on sleeping with his hat on, go with it. Remember that cognitive losses are unpredictable and inconsistent and accept even that which does not seem logical.

CARPE DIEM

Write down the single most challenging daily problem you are facing with your loved one. Is there a way to simplify the situation? For instance, lay out a towel, bathrobe and clean underwear the night before to simplify the morning routine and provide visual cues. Or, if the person wants to eat with his fingers and not a fork, don't fight it. Serve more finger food.

64.

FOCUS ON WHAT REMAINS

"What cannot be cured must be endured."

– Charlton Heston, speaking about his Alzheimer's

- People with Alzheimer's have gifts to give. Do not underestimate their strength and wisdom. They do not survive Alzheimer's without learning a thing or two.

- At every stage of the disease, there is still retained human personality, human skills, human abilities, human emotions, human communication, and the human need to be loved.

- No matter how difficult the situation may be, remember that compassionately sustaining and bearing witness to the person's ongoing life are a reflection of your humanity. By recognizing the human qualities that remain in your loved one, you show your own human virtues.

CARPE DIEM

Make a list of the human skills and abilities
that your loved one still retains.

65.

LOOK FOR SPARKS OF THE TRUE PERSON WHILE ACKNOWLEDGING THE LOSS

- Dementia is one of the greatest scourges of old age. It robs millions of older adults of their memory, reasoning, judgment, emotional stability, and use of language.

- Alzheimer's can destroy a lifetime of memories and can whittle away at the core of a person's identity. It irrevocably changes the lives of families and can exact an enormous emotional, physical, and financial toll upon caregivers.

- Yet it is important to remember that despite their losses, people with Alzheimer's retain skills and abilities. Focus on the activities that the person you love still enjoys or is capable of. Be on the watch for bits of personality that may shine through.

- For you to see and celebrate the glimmers of the real soul behind the disease, you may first need to acknowledge and mourn the losses.

CARPE DIEM

Think about your favorite parts of your loved one's personality.
Her sense of humor? His kindness? Her humility? Can
you still sometimes see these attributes you love so much,
despite the disease? Be on the watch for them today.

66.

LEARN TO PLAY AGAIN

- Play is the art of enjoying the moment with no thoughts or worries about the past or the future.

- The person with Alzheimer's may seem to be living in the past sometimes, but she may still be able to enjoy the moment if you engage her in play.

- Try simple activities that you can do together…such as swinging on a porch swing, blowing bubbles, throwing rocks into a pond, coloring with crayons, playing with a train set, etc.

- If the person with Alzheimer's is still physically robust, try more challenging play, such as tossing a Frisbee, playing croquet, riding a bike, or playing tennis. Remember, play is also good for you, so share in these playful moments.

CARPE DIEM

If circumstances allow, take the person with Alzheimer's swimming. Water play has a way of freeing the child in all of us. Community indoor pools often have very safe and friendly facilities.

67.

GET RESPITE

- Respite means a temporary reprieve, a pause from a challenging situation.

- If you are a caregiver to someone with Alzheimer's (even if it is part-time), it's important to seek out people who can help you with the care when you need a break. Your emotional, physical, social, cognitive, and spiritual health depend on it. Friends or family members are often willing to provide respite care if you only ask. Many communities offer daycare programs for people with dementia. Some communities have short-term, overnight care options. These kinds of services are often reasonably priced, with sliding-scale fees. Eldercare has a toll-free number to access local services from the Aging Resource Center or Area Agency on Aging, which can be reached at 1-800-677-1116 weekdays. They may also have suggestions about long-term care when the time comes.

- If you are not the caregiver, you may still need respite from your grief. Be sure to schedule activities you enjoy and relaxing vacations well in advance. This will give you something to look forward to.

- Remember that respite can also be found in the moment. Steal a short nap when you can. Take a quick walk in the park. Buy cut flowers and place them in a vase somewhere you'll see them often.

CARPE DIEM

Right now, take a 10-minute pause to do something
that relaxes you and that you enjoy.

68.

RECORD MEMORIES,
WHILE YOU STILL CAN

- Even when short-term memories are totally absent in a person with dementia or Alzheimer's, long-term memories often remain. In fact, sometimes memories from childhood and young adulthood seem to be sharper and more developed than they were before.

- Take this opportunity to talk to the person with Alzheimer's about his past. Ask him about his early memories. If you're specific with your questions, you might be surprised at how much detail he can retrieve. For example, ask him about elementary school. Does he remember his teachers? What did he have for lunch? Did he ever get into trouble? Who were his best friends? You might also be surprised at how much he might enjoy sharing early memories.

- If memories are bubbling up, consider recording them—either on audiotape or videotape or by writing them down. Years from now you will be glad you did.

CARPE DIEM

Buy a life history journal—the kind with blanks to fill in. There are a number out there with titles like "Memories for My Grandchild." Even if the person with Alzheimer's doesn't have grandchildren, these are excellent, simple books for capturing the unique and special life that was lived.

69.

PREPARE FOR THE SEVERE STAGE

- According to the Alzheimer's Association, there are seven stages to the disease. In the most severe stages, the devastation moves into the frontal lobes of the brain. Once the frontal lobes are damaged, the person loses the ability to interact properly. The capacity to deal with anything complicated is diminished.

- At this stage, people with Alzheimer's lose judgment, reasoning, and social skills. They may respond inappropriately and unacceptably and may have lost much of their "civilized behavior."

- If you are a caregiver, you probably can already foresee the day when you will no longer be able to care for the person at home. You may need to take the lead in making decisions regarding his welfare. In the final phases you may be dealing with finances, alternative housing, and insurance issues. Prepare the legal and financial arrangements beforehand; you will be thankful you did.

- If you are not the primary caregiver, this is one concrete and essential way that you may be able to help. Offer to assist with putting together paperwork and navigating financial challenges. Always act with respect, deference, and kindness in all of your efforts and communications. While completing paperwork such as a durable power of attorney, healthcare directives, and a will is a necessary and ultimately helpful step, it may be seen as presumptuous or "too soon." Be gentle and remember to always act in the best interests of the person with Alzheimer's as well as her caregiver.

CARPE DIEM

Have you thought through the finances and legal implications of Alzheimer's disease? Take the time to plan and prepare.

70.

RECOGNIZE THAT RESPECT AND LOVE ENDURE

- Our lives are filled with expectations and dreams of promise. Some of these dreams and expectations are fulfilled and some are not. For people with Alzheimer's and their families, friends, and caregivers, life has not turned out as expected.

- Despite this dramatic change, respect and love can endure throughout the progression of the disease. Remember that Alzheimer's may take away a person's memory but it does not take away his soul.

- In the early stages, respect and love are shown by a mother who tells her caregiving daughter her future wishes for medical treatment during the long course of the disease.

- Love is shown in the moderate stage when people who have never held a paintbrush in their lives attend Memories in the Making classes—an art project supported by the local Alzheimer's Association chapters—and create beautiful works of art that allow them to express what they are feeling.

- Respect and love are shown in the severe stage when, knowing how much his father loved the outdoors, a son pushes his father's bed out onto the patio on sunny days, even though his dad can no longer express his wishes. Communication and love do not always need words.

CARPE DIEM

Think about your loved one's present condition. How can you communicate love and respect today, not only with your words but with your actions?

LIVE WITH MEANING AND PURPOSE

Even as you grieve, mourn, and perhaps care for the person with Alzheimer's, you can live a life of meaning and purpose. The trick is in getting in touch with your innermost self—the part that knows why you were put here on Earth and what really matters to you. After all, grief and love are inseparable twins—the yin and yang of life.

71.

KEEP YOUR SENSE OF HUMOR

"Now I'm one of the few men who will ask for directions."

– a man with early-stage Alzheimer's and a sense of humor

- Humor can help you get through many crises. Try to see the light side of what is happening. Appreciate the humor in daily foibles and don't become so overly serious that you lose your zest for life.

- Build humor into your daily schedule. Watch your favorite late-night talk show or program on Comedy Central. Read the funnies. Find funny videos on YouTube. Whatever makes you laugh out loud—do that. Every day.

- Remember that the person with dementia is still a person. He needs a good laugh too. Those with Alzheimer's can maintain their sense of humor well into the disease. Relive a funny occurrence from your mutual past and share a laugh.

- Sharing your experiences with other families affected by Alzheimer's may be helpful as well to let you see the humor still in your lives. Surprisingly, members of these groups often find their shared experiences funny as well as sad.

CARPE DIEM

Who is your funniest friend, neighbor, or family member?
Call this person or spend a few minutes with him today.

72.

HEAD TOWARDS A NEW NORMAL

"Always remember that the future comes one day at a time."

— Dean Acheson

- A diagnosis of early Alzheimer's accompanies changes in thinking, mood, and performance that both you and your loved one probably have noticed for a while. These changes may have been frightening and frustrating to both of you.

- But even after the diagnosis, the person you love is still the same person. There is just a better understanding of what is going on within his brain.

- The trick is staying flexible and blame-free. Right now you are adapting to a chronic condition and in effect creating a new "normal."

- Try to keep in mind that "normal" is relative. What was normal before doesn't work anymore, so it's time for a new one. Change can be hard, but try to roll with the punches.

CARPE DIEM

Resilience is the term that psychologists use to talk about a person's capacity to change and adapt with ease. Today, talk to someone whom you have observed has been especially resilient to life changes. Ask her how she does it.

73.

PRACTICE A TRANSFORMATIONAL COPING STYLE

- If you can take charge of your life and begin to feel in control again, you can withstand an enormous amount of change and even thrive on the stress. On the other hand, if you keep yourself in a helpless position, you will find it hard to cope.

- Developing an "attitude of hardiness," described by psychologists as a transformational coping style, can be helpful during times of crisis and loss. People who refuse to see themselves as victims and transform the challenging experience of dealing with Alzheimer's into opportunity get through the crisis with greater ease.

- People with this transformational coping style believe they can influence events and tend to approach change as an opportunity for personal growth. By contrast, people who lack this attitude of hardiness often view themselves as helpless. They get lost in their emotional reactions, withdraw from others, and have little motivation to do anything about their problems.

- The good news is that you can choose to use this transformational approach while coping with the losses of Alzheimer's. This coping style can help move you from feelings of helplessness to experiencing a greater sense of control.

- No matter how disruptive this diagnosis has been, it can be transformed into an experience that leaves you wiser and more capable of building something entirely new out of your life.

CARPE DIEM

What worrisome thoughts about dealing with Alzheimer's are bothering you? Write these down. What are the possible solutions to these problems? What opportunities are there to transform these worries into something new and inviting for your life? If you're better at thinking aloud than on paper, talk through these ideas with a friend.

74.

ADVOCATE

- Consider honoring the person with Alzheimer's through social activism. The local or regional branch of the Alzheimer's Association probably organizes a fundraising walk you could participate in.

- Write letters to your elected officials persuading them to support families affected by Alzheimer's through legislative action.

- You might also consider volunteering for a different cause, perhaps one that was near and dear to the person with Alzheimer's.

- Many grieving people find that they get much more out of their volunteer efforts than they put in. And volunteering is also a way of affirming the preciousness of life.

- If your schedule is too hectic, offer money instead of time. Make your donation in honor of the person with Alzheimer's.

CARPE DIEM

Visit alz.org and click on Advocate.

75.

FINISH SOMETHING, AS A GIFT

- The person with dementia or Alzheimer's may have had a dream or goal that she was unable to finish because of the disease's progress. Could you finish it for her?

- This could be something substantial—like adding a deck to the back of the house—or simple—like organizing family photos.

- Get others to pitch in and help you complete this task. You will find that people often have a hard time knowing how they can help, but when you ask them to do something tangible and specific, they'll jump right in.

- When the task is complete, tell the person with Alzheimer's about it. Invite everyone who participated and have a little celebration. Take photos and share them.

CARPE DIEM

Call up someone else who cares about the person with Alzheimer's and brainstorm a list of possible tasks to complete.

76.

TAKE A RISK

- Sometimes it takes something as bracing as a loved one's dementia diagnosis to awaken us to life's true potential. To our *own* true potential.

- What have you always wanted to do but never have? What have you always wanted to try but have been too afraid?

- There's no time like the present. In fact, there is ever only the present.

- If you're fearful, start with a small risk…something where the consequences are insignificant. Take that singing lesson you've always wanted to take. What's the worst that could happen…the singing instructor doesn't think you're the next Pavarotti?

- Work your way up to something big.

CARPE DIEM

Make a list of at least 100 things that you've always wanted to be, do, or have. Pick one and take one small step toward it today.

77.

DISCOVER YOUR CALLING

- We believe that we were put here on Earth for a reason. For me (Alan), it was to help others mourn well so they can go on to live and love well. For me (Kirby), it was to help people be their physical best so they can be as happy and fulfilled as possible.

- We believe that you have a calling too. What is it? Keep in mind that it's not always a "job" (although if you can get paid to do your calling, that's the best case scenario!). It might be a volunteer or caretaking role.

- If you haven't yet discovered your calling, now's the time. You probably have a sense of what it is, but you may need to try volunteering or shadowing others to figure it out.

- If you have discovered your calling, excellent. Make sure you're spending your days doing what matters most to you.

- If you're the primary caregiver to the person with Alzheimer's and have had to put your calling on hold for now, try to stay connected to it through reading and participating in online groups.

CARPE DIEM

What was the calling of the person with Alzheimer's? Choose
a symbol of that calling and give it to him as a gift.

78.

LEARN TO MEDITATE

- Deep breathing and meditation can change your life. The benefits are physical, emotional, and spiritual. Meditation invites your body into a more relaxed physical state, more restful sleep, lowers your blood pressure, increases oxygen circulation, improves your immune system, increases your ability to concentrate, calms your mind, and stimulates an overall feeling of well-being.

- Give yourself five full minutes to concentrate on your breathing. Breathe from your diaphragm; push your stomach out as you breathe in and pull your stomach in as you breathe out. Imagine that you're inhaling the spiritual energy you need to help you integrate loss into your life and that you're exhaling your feelings of sadness and grief. No, this doesn't make your grief go away, but it helps soothe your soul.

- Breathing opens you up. Grief may have naturally closed you down. The power of breath helps to fill your empty spaces. The old wisdom of "count to ten" is all about taking a breath to open up space for something to happen. The paradox is that in slowing down, you create divine momentum that invites you to continue to mourn.

- There are many resources available to help you learn how to meditate. One of my personal favorites is a classic simply titled *How to Meditate*, by Lawrence LeShan (Bantam Books, available in paperback).

CARPE DIEM

Make a commitment right now to learn how to meditate. Pick up the book noted above within the next three days. Just a few minutes of meditation each day will provide you a wonderful spiritual perspective on where you are in your life's journey.

79.

SPEND TIME WITH A PET

- Pets can be a wonderful source of comfort during times of grief. You can be needy, depressed, confused—and your pets still love you. They don't pressure you to "keep busy" or "carry on;" they don't ask you to "let go of" or "resolve" your grief. Your pets love you regardless of your weight, haircut, or body shape. Yes, your pets love you without judgment. And you feel that love and appreciate its steadfast presence in your life. Unlike many things in life, with a pet you comparatively give so little and get so much back in return.

- People with Alzheimer's also often find great joy and comfort from the company of a pet.

- We pet lovers sometimes call our pets "companion animals" because they are in fact our companions. Not only can pets be your companions, but they can also help meet your need for physical contact. As you touch your pet, you are comforted, calmed, and grounded.

- Caring for and enjoying the company of animals—dogs, cats, horses, birds, deer, even fish—can offer an abundant supply of solace that many medical studies have found can help you live a longer and healthier life. Giving your attention to animals also requires you to slow down, be quiet, and become more aware of your environment. That, in turn, leads to a renewed sense of wonder and gratitude for the marvels that the world contains.

CARPE DIEM

If you have a pet, spend extra time with her today. If you don't, arrange to borrow an animal from a friend for the day.

80.

KNOW THAT YOU ARE LOVED

- As Jane Howard wisely observed, "Call it a clan, call it a network, call it a tribe, call it a family. Whatever you call it, whoever you are, you need one." Yes, love from family, friends, and community gives life meaning and purpose. Look around for expressions of care and concern. These are people who love you and want to be an important part of your support system.

- Some of those who love you may not know how to reach out to you, but they still love you. Reflect on the people who care about you and the ways in which your life matters. Open your heart and have gratitude for those who love you.

- Feeling connected to people around you can be a great source of joy and a cause for celebration. When you reach out to others, and they to you, you remember you are loved even during days of darkness and grief. When you consciously come together with family, friends and community, you make the most of each moment and experience a sense of well-being and belonging in the world.

- It is vital to create a sense of community that is spiritually nurturing and responsive to the needs surrounding loss in your life. Your relationships with family, friends, and community are connected like a circle, with no end and no beginning. When you allow yourself to be a part of that circle, you find your place. You realize you belong and are a vital part of a bigger whole.

CARPE DIEM

Get out some notes and cards you have received from
people who care about you. Re-read them and remind
yourself that you are loved. Then, call someone you love
and express gratitude that she or he is in your life.

81.

ALLOW GOD TO SPEAK TO YOU

- We hear so much about praying to God, but what about allowing God to speak to you?

- In the Bible, the book of Exodus chronicles the story of God delivering his people, the Israelites, from the bondage of slavery. Those of you who have not read the book of Exodus may be familiar with the epic film *The Ten Commandments*, in which a young Charlton Heston plays the role of Moses.

- Exodus Chapter 3 picks up the story with a young shepherd named Moses tending a flock of sheep. While tending the flock, Moses comes across a strange sight. He encounters a bush that is on fire but does not burn up. His curiosity gets the better of him so he wanders over to get a closer look. It is there that he encounters the presence of God, and it is there that Moses hears God's plan for a suffering nation.

- Our mourning experiences touch us in profound ways at the very core of our body, mind, and soul. Lamenting can be a result of intense suffering; it is our way of communicating with God.

- But Moses also shows us that God communicates with us. You may not find God in a burning bush, but you may find Him in the stillness of the moment, in the wind, in the natural world that surrounds us. Yes, God speaks to us if we take the time to listen.

CARPE DIEM

Seek out those quiet, still places and listen to God's voice.
Open yourself to the verse "Be still and know that I
am God." And remember that one of the final things
God said to Moses was, "I will be with you."

82.

BEAUTIFY YOUR ENVIRONMENT

- Many people believe that not only does the environment in which you live influence the way you think and feel, it is a reflection of the way you think and feel.

- How does your home environment mirror your inner life? Are they both chaotic, cluttered, ill-cared for? Read a bit about the principles of feng shui.

- First, de-clutter. Ask a friend or family member to help you. Complete one room at a time. If you are the primary caregiver to the person with Alzheimer's, decluttering will help him too.

- Next, clean, or hire someone to clean. Either way, it's worth it.

- Now, freshen up the room with new paint, window coverings, pillows, etc. Hire a decorator for a one-hour consultation if you need help with this step.

- Finally, sit in your newly beautified room and relax. Notice how the room's energy affects your energy.

CARPE DIEM

Start small. De-clutter one drawer or one closet today. After,
see how the newly organized space makes you feel.

83.

LIVE WITH PURPOSE

- Do you believe things happen for a reason? Do you think you attract what you are thinking about?

- You may not be sold 100 percent on the popular notion of the power of attraction, but you will notice that if you live your life with awareness and intention, you are living your life in the best possible manner.

- If you set your intention to heal the losses you have felt from your loved one's Alzheimer's and to enjoy the human traits he still possesses, then, despite the pain of the losses, you are living your life with purpose. You are living with the awareness that your intentional thoughts can create, to some extent, your own destiny.

- Your life is a miracle. Your loved one's life is a miracle. Live your lives with the awe and wonder that they deserve. Enjoy each other and each day and live with purpose.

CARPE DIEM

Today, set your intention for the coming year. With what attitude do you intend to live each day? How do you intend to mourn your losses? How can you embrace the human qualities of the person you love and live well again?

84.

BEFRIEND EIGHT UNIVERSAL HEALING PRINCIPLES

• Eight healing principles, used in the majority of cultures, can help sustain your physical, emotional, cognitive, social, and spiritual well-being. Explore the list below and note which of the universal principles you are embracing and which you are neglecting.

Support health and well-being	Non-supportive of health and well-being
Balanced diet	Unbalanced diet
Daily and weekly exercise	Lack of exercise
Time for fun, play, and laughter	Loss of humor and lack of fun and play
Music, sonics, and chanting	Lack of music, sonics, and chanting
Love, touch, and support systems	Lack of love, touch, and support systems
Engaged in interests, hobbies, and creative purpose	Lack of interests, hobbies, and creative purpose
Nature, beauty, and healing environments	Lack of nature, beauty, and healing environments
Faith and belief in the supernatural	Lack of faith and belief in the supernatural

CARPE DIEM

Make a commitment to rebalance those areas that are not supportive to your overall well-being. Get out a piece of paper right now and write out an "action plan for creating balance."

85.

REDEFINE SUCCESS

- Success in loving someone with Alzheimer's is expressing that love. It is continuing to find ways and moments in which to enjoy your relationship.

- Success is helping the person with Alzheimer's retain, for as long as possible, his values and purpose in life, and of course, his sense of self. If he is lucky, his sense of humor will continue to find expression in his new life.

- Is this a fantasy, to still feel successful? No, it can happen. We know that any disease that gets worse over time requires people to face uncertainty, grieve, and adapt to new losses. We know that the embarrassment caused by a "senior moment" differs greatly from the frustration and fear caused by the memory problems of Alzheimer's, but we also know that people can adapt and endure with grace.

CARPE DIEM

Try something new with your loved one today. Consider
art, dancing, or walking in the park. Or ask her what
she has always wanted to do but has never tried.

86.

DO WHAT YOU LOVE

- You've heard the expression, "Do what you love and the rest will follow."

- When your life is challenged by Alzheimer's, you need to simplify, so we're simplifying this saying to, "Do what you love." Period. There's no "rest," no "more" that is required.

- If you are a caregiver to the person with Alzheimer's, having the freedom to do what you love may be difficult or impossible right now. Travel, for example, may be out of the question. OK…what else do you love? What did you love as a child that you have forgotten about? What hopes and dreams that you had set aside could you now explore? What little things that give you pleasure could you integrate into your day? (Think things like fresh flowers, a cup of hot tea with honey, a bubble bath, the latest novel by your favorite author, a phone call to your grandchild.)

- If you are not the primary caregiver, you may feel guilty about doing what you love. Why should you get to have all the fun while the person with Alzheimer's and the caregiver are so stuck? Well, you may be able to help with the caregiving. But you are also responsible to yourself, to make God smile at what you do with your life.

- Similarly, find ways to increase the amount of time that the person you care about spends doing what he enjoys. Your loved one may surprise you in what he still can do, giving you back the lasting gift of memories.

CARPE DIEM

Today, spend at least 15 minutes doing something that
you love that you haven't done for a long, long time.

87.

PAY ATTENTION TO SYNCHRONICITIES

- Stuff happens, the saying goes. (Well, you know the real saying…)

- The philosophy embedded in that aphorism is that things happen over which you have no control, and you need to resign yourself to the fact that life is often painful.

- Sometimes life *is* painful. Sometimes stuff happens. But often, if you are paying attention, if you are living on purpose, stuff happens that is nothing short of miraculous.

- At night you dream of a friend you haven't seen for years, and the next day she calls you, out of the blue. You hear a song on the car radio that perfectly captures what you're feeling that moment. Your furnace breaks down and you receive an unexpected check in the mail.

- Pay attention to coincidences. Believe that they may be telling you something—even guiding you. As the Dalai Lama said, "I am open to the guidance of synchronicity and do not let expectations hinder my path."

CARPE DIEM

The next time you experience what feels like a coincidence, write it down on your calendar. Contemplate what guidance it may be offering.

88.

SHOW YOUR TRUE GRIT

"When tragedy strikes, most of us ultimately rebound surprisingly well. Where does this resilience come from?"

– Gary Stix from *The Neuroscience of True Grit*

• Convention, at least in the past, has held that psychological resilience to life's stresses was a fairly rare event, a product of lucky genes or good parenting. But research into bereavement and natural disasters has found in recent years that the trait of resilience is, in fact, relatively commonplace.

• People respond to the worst life has to offer with a variety of behaviors, some of which might seem narcissistic or dysfunctional at another time. But it is these behaviors—coping ugly, as one researcher calls it—that ultimately help us adapt in a crisis.

• Resilience begins at a primal level. If you want to know the biology of it, in crisis, the hypothalamus, which is a relay station in our brains, churns out signals that release stress hormones. Certain protective biochemicals help resilient people switch these signals back off.

• However, not everyone can rebound this way. In fact, about 10 percent of those facing emotional trauma get mired in anxiety and depression and may need to see a counselor or physician in order to bounce back.

• The lesson here is that you need to find what works for you. What will allow you to muddle through the crisis of navigating Alzheimer's? The odds are good you have the true grit that will allow you to do this on your own. If not, then help is readily available.

CARPE DIEM

Think about what works for you when you're under stress. Do you need to step away? Do you need to focus on your own needs for a while before you can help others? Figure out which "coping ugly" strategies work for you. Find your true grit.

89.

RE-EXAMINE YOUR PRIORITIES

- Seeing a tragic disease like Alzheimer's has a way of making us rethink our lives and the meaningfulness of how we spend them. It tends to awaken us to what is truly important in our lives.

- What gives your life meaning? What doesn't? Take steps to spend more of your time on what is meaningful and less on what is not.

- Now could be the time for you to reconfigure your life. Begin volunteering. Share with other Alzheimer's families. Open yourself up to new possibilities, new relationships. Help others in regular, ongoing ways. Move closer to your family members.

- After dealing with life crises like Alzheimer's, many people can no longer stand to be around people who seem shallow, egocentric, or mean-spirited. It is OK to let these so-called friends go. Instead, find ways to connect with people who share your new outlook on life, and live your life with meaning.

CARPE DIEM

Make a list with two columns: What's important to me. What's not. Spend at least 15 minutes brainstorming and writing.

90.

EXERCISE YOUR BRAIN

- You've seen enough of dementia or Alzheimer's up close to hope it doesn't happen to anyone else you love—or to you.

- Researchers think that activities that exercise your brain, such as math and crossword puzzles, may help stave off dementia.

- A famous ongoing Alzheimer's study—called the Nun Study for short, because its subjects are 678 Sisters at a convent in Minnesota—has shown that richer language skills are linked with lower susceptibility to Alzheimer's. So tasks such as reading and writing may be preventive.

- We still don't know enough about Alzheimer's disease to know for sure what causes it or how to prevent it…but we have some good clues. You're reading a book right now, so you're on the right track.

CARPE DIEM

What kind of brain puzzles or tasks do you most enjoy? Get a stack of them and place a few everywhere you sit in your house as well as in our car (great while you wait for an appointment).

91.

ACKNOWLEDGE YOUR CLOUD OF WITNESSES

- The Bible says that we are preceded and surrounded by a cloud of witnesses.

- Those whom we have loved and who have gone before us now serve as our witnesses. We like to think that they watch us with great fondness, forgiving our foibles and rejoicing in our kindnesses—and looking forward to the day when we will join them.

- Among our cloud of witnesses are untold others who also struggled with the illness of someone loved, who also despaired in the "dark night of the soul." Some of the more learned and eloquent of these people wrote books about their experiences with despair and finding hope again. You might be helped by reading the writings of witnesses such as Henri Nouwen, C.S. Lewis, and Catherine Marshall.

- Our cloud of witnesses also includes the great world and spiritual leaders who have shaped the course of history. Just think…what if Jesus and the Buddha and Lao Tzu are all hanging out together, watching us right now. What are they saying to each other?

CARPE DIEM

Pretend you could have dinner tonight with seven of the people in your cloud of witnesses. Who would you choose and why?

92.

REACH OUT AND TOUCH

- For many people, physical contact with another human being is healing. It has been recognized since ancient times as having transformative, healing powers.

- Have you hugged anyone lately? Held someone's hand? Put your arm around another human being?

- You probably know several people who enjoy hugging or physical touching. If you're comfortable with their touch, encourage it in the weeks and months to come.

- The person who has dementia may still enjoy your touch. Hold his hand. Give him a backrub. Comb his hair.

- You may want to listen to the song titled, "I Know What Love Is," by Don White. I have found this song helps me reflect on the power of touch. Listen to this song then drop Alan a note or e-mail (drwolfelt@centerforloss.com) and let me know how it makes you think, and more important, feel.

CARPE DIEM

Try hugging your close friends and family members today, even if you usually don't. You just might like it!

93.

LOOK FOR THE SURPRISES
AND GIFTS IN YOUR DAY

- Stop reading this and look around you where you are right this moment. Look at the same things you see each day, but through a different set of eyes. What are you grateful for that is within your view? See it with awe. Look at the face of the person with Alzheimer's and rejoice that he is still in your life, despite the challenges.

- Whatever comes into your path today, consider it a gift. Take a moment to receive the gift and appreciate the giver. Embrace the warm feelings that come from being connected, from the link to gratefulness. Say "yes" and "thank you."

- Bill Keane said, "Yesterday's the past, tomorrow's the future, but today is a gift. That's why it's called the present."

CARPE DIEM

Create a "Surprises and Gifts" Journal. Keep a running list of what you are thankful for, the surprises that come to you each day, and the gifts you receive. Be specific: I am thankful for the gift of the gorgeous blue sky, the smile on my neighbor's face.

94.

ADD MEANING TO YOUR DAYS

- You may have already taken up the mantra of "Don't sweat the small stuff," which is essential in dealing with Alzheimer's. But also don't ignore the "big stuff," like friends, forgiveness, and faith. Get the big stuff in order and with a little planning and help, and maybe a little nudging, the rest will fall into place.

- Be sure you've addressed the following issues:

  - Find someone to confide in. This can be someone from an Alzheimer's support group or a close friend.
  - Learn to forgive. Everyone, including you, your relatives, other family members, friends, and doctors, will make mistakes. Forgive others for disappointing you, but also forgive yourself if you feel you have made mistakes.
  - Set limits. If you feel exhausted, lower your expectations and re-examine your priorities. Be willing to say, "Sorry, I can't" more often.
  - Take comfort in your spiritual beliefs and moral values. Your spiritual feelings and faith may deepen as you continue to care for your loved one.
  - Don't miss out on a minute to relax. There is an exhausting amount of busyness that can fill your day. Take mini-breaks when you can. Take a moment outside to read the paper in the sunshine when you pick it up. Put some relaxing music on while making dinner. Peek at the stars when you let the cat out. You deserve it.

CARPE DIEM

What "big stuff" have you struggled to deal with? Finding someone to talk to? Forgiving yourself and others? Setting limits? Taking care of your spiritual needs? Taking care of yourself? Make a list of what you might do to move forward and take care of the "big stuff" in your life.

95.

KEEP HOPE IN YOUR HEART

"There is no medicine like hope, no incentive so great and no tonic so powerful as the expectation of something better tomorrow."

– Orison Marden

- How can one have hope when you are dealing with an incurable disease? Well, it depends on what you are hoping *for*. It's true that a cure for Alzheimer's does not appear to be in sight. But life is not infinite for any of us. In fact, none of us will get out of this life alive.

- But, we can still have hope about how we live our lives. Alzheimer's may take away memory, but it cannot take away our hope to enjoy the time we have here on earth with our loved ones.

- Remember, life gives us brief moments with the ones we love. But sometimes in those moments we create memories that can last a lifetime.

- Live your life, moment by moment, filled with hope, and you will create memories that will fill your life and your loved ones' too.

CARPE DIEM

What is it that you hope for in the time you have left on earth with your loved one? Fill your life with hope, and take steps to enjoy the time you have.

96.

RECOGNIZE THE DUAL
ASPECT OF CHANGE

- The Chinese symbol for change is a combination of the symbols for crisis and opportunity. Change not only brings a feeling of crisis but also opens opportunity for you to look at the basis of your life, why you are here, and what you want to do with the rest of your life.

- Thus change has a dual identity. Even as you experience the searing pain of the losses Alzheimer's brings, it is important to recognize that there IS opportunity in this experience. There is the possibility that by caring and being genuinely kind and human with one another, that you will not only grow as a person, but that you can help to spread kindness in the world.

- It may sound odd to say there is opportunity in Alzheimer's, but if you open yourself to transforming your life, you will find new opportunities to explore, opportunities that will help you move toward creating the life that you desire.

- By helping those around you, you are really helping yourself to understand the sanctity of life. Make a point each day to be sure you are doing the things in your life that are important to you.

CARPE DIEM

Take the opportunity to look at your life and write down what you consider to be the 10 most important activities that you engage in regularly. Now write down next to each how much of your time you spend doing these important things. If you are not spending much time on those important things, take the opportunity to change that.

97.

FORGIVE

- You may be harboring some spiteful feelings. Perhaps you are angry at a medical caregiver. Maybe you're upset at friends and family who haven't been there for you in your time of need. Maybe you are mad at the person with Alzheimer's.

- Forgiveness is an act of surrender. If you surrender your resentment, you are freeing yourself of a very heavy load. You are surrendering your human feelings of judgment to the only One who is truly in a position to judge. Don't go to your own grave angry.

- Forgive. Write letters of forgiveness if this will help you unburden yourself, even if you never send the letters.

- And while you're at it, don't forget to forgive yourself. Self-recrimination is negative energy. If you did something wrong, acknowledge, apologize, and forgive.

- This Idea calls to mind this poem by William Arthur Ward, an American pastor and teacher:

Before you speak, listen.
Before you write, think.
Before you spend, earn.
Before you invest, investigate.
Before you criticize, wait.
Before you pray, forgive.
Before you quit, try.
Before you retire, save.
Before you die, give.

CARPE DIEM

Today, call or stop by to visit someone you've been holding a grudge against. Tell this person you've missed her company and would like to catch up.

98.

IMAGINE THE PERSON WITH ALZHEIMER'S IN HEAVEN

- Do you believe in an afterlife? Many mourners I have had the honor of companioning in their journeys are comforted by a belief or a hope that somehow, somewhere, their loved ones who grow ill and eventually die live on after death in health and happiness. For some, this belief is anchored in a religious faith. For others, it is simply a spiritual sense.

- If you do believe in an afterlife, you might take comfort in thinking about your loved one being restored to full health and happiness. This is not to hasten his death, of course, or to squander the time you have left together, but rather to have hope for the far-off future.

- You might find it healing to write a poem or a story or draw a picture of what the Heaven you imagine is like. Or you could create a collage. Cut out images from magazines and/or scrapbooking supplies that convey the look and feel of your Heaven, and assemble them together on a piece of poster board. Whenever your heart is heavy, spend a minute or two seeking solace in your Heavenly collage.

CARPE DIEM

Close your eyes right now and imagine what Heaven might be like. See the person you love no longer sick but instead vigorous and smiling. Perhaps that is the happy end of the long and arduous road you are now walking.

99.

LIVE WITH GRATITUDE AND COUNT YOUR BLESSINGS

"Well, Susan has done it again. A piece of her artwork has been picked by the judges to be in the Alzheimer's Memories in the Making program. This is quite an honor for Susan and her memory. I am very proud of her."

– email from a patient whose wife passed away from Alzheimer's

- When you are faced with a horrible disease like Alzheimer's and feel the slow loss of the person you love, it can be difficult to have a sense of gratitude about your life, yet gratitude prepares you for the blessings yet to come.

- Many blessings have already been companioning you since you started on the Alzheimer's journey with your loved one. Somehow, and with grace, you have survived. Think back and recognize the many supportive gestures, big and small, you have already been offered along the way. Recognize that even when your loved one is gone, you will continue to receive blessings from the memories you have shared.

- When you fill your life with gratitude, you invoke a self-fulfilling prophecy. What you expect to happen *can* happen. If you anticipate support and nurturance, you will find it. If you don't expect anyone to support you, often they don't.

- Think of all that you have to be thankful for. This is not to minimize the difficulty of your present situation, but to allow you to reflect on the possibilities for love and joy each day. Honor those possibilities and have gratitude for them. Be grateful for your physical health and strong spirit. Be grateful for your family and friends and the time you can still share with the person you love. Above all, be grateful for this very moment. When you are grateful, you prepare the way for inner peace.

CARPE DIEM

Start keeping a gratitude journal. Each night before bed, record the blessings from the day. At first this may seem challenging, but if you continue the daily practice, it will get easier and more joyful.

100.

REMEMBER THAT LOVE LIVES ON

"Love bears all things, believes all things, hopes all things, endures all things."

— 1 Corinthians 13:7

- It's worrisome to think about the failing memory of the person with Alzheimer's and that at some point in the future, she may no longer remember or even recognize you as a person she loves. Will her love be able to endure the ravages of Alzheimer's? Can she really still love you if she can't even recognize you?

- It's a shock to most people when they are no longer recognized, and it is hard not to feel pain and offense when this happens. But it's important to reframe this experience and remember that it is the disease that has caused this state of affairs, not the person.

- Try to remember that it is the person's brain that has been ravaged by the disease, not his heart. And even though he may be confused and not even recognize you, in his heart there is still love for you and for the care and love you have given him.

- Do you believe that there is a soul that transcends the physical body? Many people believe that the brain is the control room of the physical body, but it is not the seat of the soul. Therefore that which is eternal and divine in the person you love lives on, unharmed by the disease. And that is where his love for you lives, too.

CARPE DIEM

If you have kept any old letters or birthday cards the person with Alzheimer's sent you in the past, get them out today and spend some time immersing yourself in his love for you.

A FINAL WORD

"People think it's a terrible tragedy when somebody has Alzheimer's. But in my mother's case, it's different. My mother has been unhappy all of her life. For the first time in her life, she is happy."

– Amy Tan

Alzheimer's disease affects each person uniquely. Generally it is a tragic disease, and the losses its victims and their friends and family suffer are tremendous.

We hope that this book has helped you acknowledge that when you care about someone who has been diagnosed with dementia or Alzheimer's disease, you suffer losses long before the person's death. These losses, like the disease itself, are ambiguous and progressive.

We grieve and we grieve and we grieve as we watch the inexorable progress of this brain-changing disease. As it advances, much of your treasured life together is lost, as the memories of your shared past get trapped in the faulty circuits of your loved one's brain.

On your journey through Alzheimer's disease, we encourage you to recognize your losses, embrace your feelings about them, and outwardly mourn them in ways that are comfortable to you. You must let your grief out. Mourning allows the darkness of your internal grieving to come out into the light and be released from the depths of your soul. To emerge from the darkness of Alzheimer's grief, you must mourn to enter the light—and to re-enter your life.

We also hope you are coming to see that to stay close to your loved one as her brain disease progresses, you must emphasize the abilities she retains and seek to join her, wherever she is. No one can stop this disease—not the person affected, not science, not medicine, not you. Remember the words of Ronald Reagan, one of the most famous Alzheimer's victims:

"You know, people get frustrated because their loved ones who have Alzheimer's, 'Oh, he doesn't recognize me anymore, how can I recognize this person, if they don't recognize me? They're not the same person.' Well, they are the same person, but they have a brain disease. And it is not their fault they have this disease."

Your loved one truly is still the same person, but a disease is robbing him of the brain circuits that once made his life more complete. Now there are injuries and gaps in his functioning. But things will not be made better by dwelling on the gaps or the deterioration of behavior. Emphasize the positive and join him in art, in singing, in remembering the good times, in whatever he can still do. He is still the person you love.

Finally, invite hope into your journey through Alzheimer's. No, there is no cure on the horizon for this devastating disease. But if you mourn your losses and move towards a life of meaning and purpose, your remaining days with your loved one can still be full of special moments, new memories, and even fulfillment in your relationship. Remember that your loved one still loves you. Love is not a function of the brain. It cannot be eliminated by a brain disease. Faulty chemicals and circuits in the brain cannot affect love. Love is in our hearts and in our souls. Love endures.

SEND US YOUR IDEAS FOR HEALING GRIEF CAUSED BY ALZHEIMER'S

We'd love to hear your practical ideas forhealing your grieving heart when someone you care about has Alzheimer's. We may use them in other books someday. Please jot down your idea and mail it to:

Center for Loss and Life Transition
3735 Broken Bow Road
Fort Collins, CO 80526
Or email us at DrWolfelt@centerforloss.com
or go to this website, www.centerforloss.com.

We hope to hear from you!

My idea:

_____

_____

_____

_____

_____

_____

My name and mailing address:

_____

_____

_____

_____